KT-371-453

MASSAGE

for common ailments

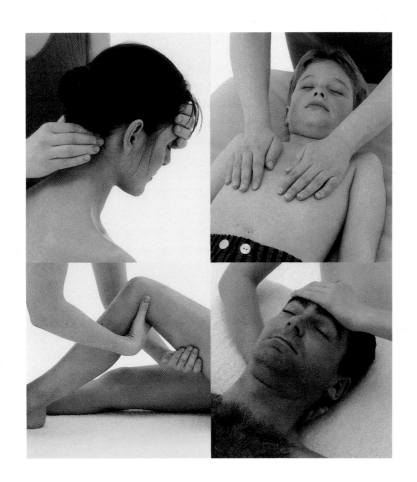

MASSAGE
for common ailments

PENNY RICH

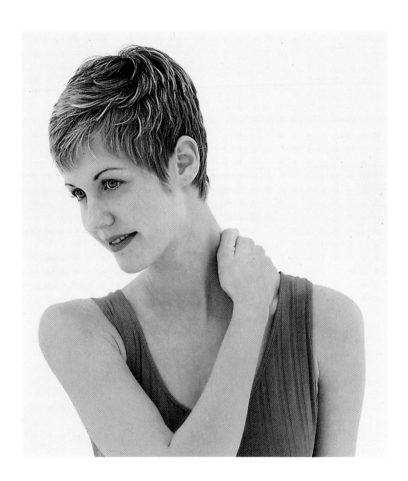

•PARRAGON•

WARNING

If you have a medical condition, or are pregnant, the massages described in this book should not be followed without consulting your doctor first. All guidelines, warnings and massage captions should be read carefully *before* embarking on any of the massages.
The publisher cannot accept responsibility for injuries or damage arising out of a failure to comply with the above.

PICTURE CREDITS:

PWA International: 8, 11, 18, 30, 36, 48, 60, 92, 104
Spectrum Colour Library: 86
Tony Stone Images: 110; /Leslie Sponseller: 42; /Andre Perlstein: 54; /Bruce Ayres: 66;
/Chris Harvey: 76; /Julian Calder: 118
ZEFA: 24, 72, 82, 98, 122
Every effort has been made to trace the copyright holders and we apologise in advance for any unintentional omissions. We would be pleased to insert the appropriate acknowledgement in any subsequent edition of this publication.

First published in Great Britain in 1994 by
Parragon Book Service Ltd
Unit 13-17 Avonbridge Trading Estate
Atlantic Road, Avonmouth
Bristol BS11 9QD

This edition published in 1996

Copyright © Parragon Book Service Ltd 1994

All rights reserved.
No part of this publication may be reproduced, stored in a retrieval system or transmitted in any form by any means electronic, mechanical, photocopying or otherwise without first obtaining written permission of the copyright holder.

ISBN 0 75251 934 4

Editorial: Linda Doeser Publishing Services
Design and DTP: Kingfisher Design Services, London
Step-by-step photography: Susanna Price

Printed in Great Britain

CONTENTS

THE MIRACLE OF MASSAGE

One of the best things about massage is that anyone can do it. It is so easy that you can learn the basic strokes in a single session. It is the one therapy where you do not have to be an expert – you can just feel your way as it is based on the natural human instinct to soothe and comfort someone by touch. It needs no fancy equipment – just a pair of hands and some oil. Moreover, it is the quickest, simplest, most pleasurable and inexpensive way to make someone healthier and happier.

Massage is also one of the best ways to treat many of our commonest modern-day ailments. Problems such as stress, lack of energy, Repetitive Strain Injury, sleeplessness, fatigue, PMT, cellulite, headache, back ache, tummy ache and, in fact, any aches or pains anywhere in the body, feel instantly better after the right massage routine.

This is not just wishful thinking from a lot of cranks who like to believe that massage cures everything. Medical scientists studying massage have proved that it is a natural tranquillizer. Indeed, stroking the body slows the heartbeat and lowers blood pressure and this is the fastest and most effective way to relax. As research now shows that stress and sickness go hand in hand, the more relaxed you are, the healthier you will be.

Its worth as a natural pain-reliever has been proved throughout time. Ever since Stone Age man patted his pet mammoth, touch has calmed the savage beast in us all. In fact, even though you are probably not aware of it, you use it every day whenever you rub a hurt elbow, stroke tired eyes to stop them aching, or cuddle a crying baby and pat his back to relieve wind.

(Right) Massage is the quickest, surest way to create a sense of well-being.

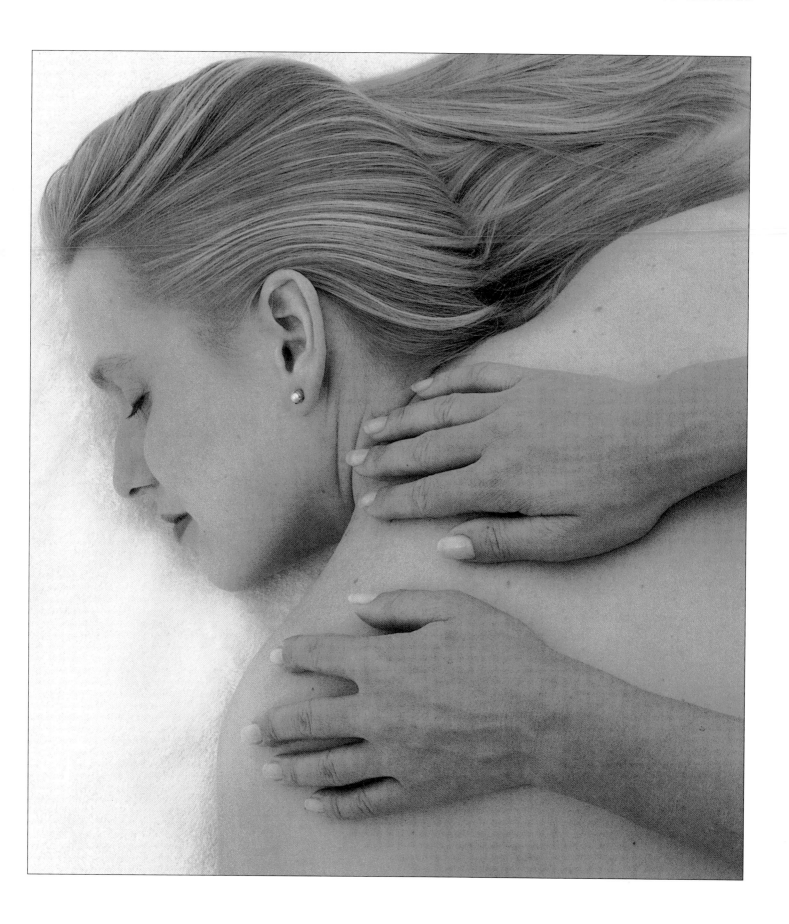

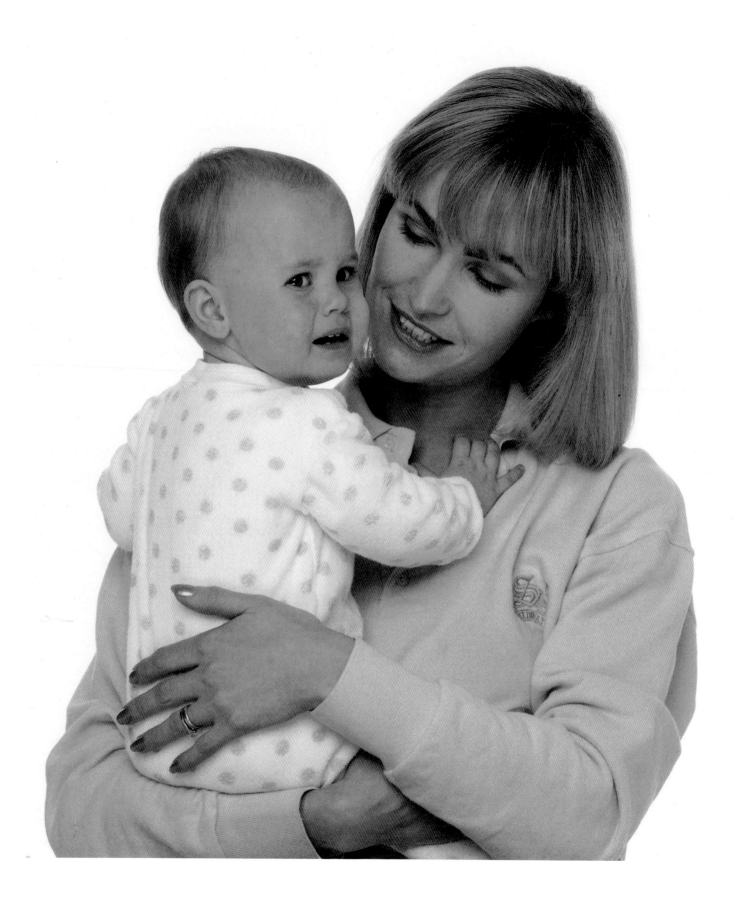

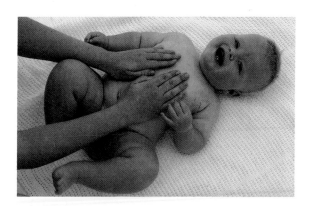

Touch does more than just get rid of pain – it is also comforting, soothing, reassuring, pampering and, above all, it makes you feel happy. This is the real miracle of massage – the fact that it soothes both mind and body in a single stroke – and that something as simple as rubbing skin against skin can make you feel better in minutes, rather than days, weeks or months.

Massage can work miracles on a grander scale, too. Used therapeutically, in physiotherapy for instance, it can help the disabled become stronger. It is an effective way of getting emotionally disturbed patients to relax and talk to therapists. Studies in intensive care wards of hospitals show that people in coma recover quicker if they are touched, stroked and cuddled. Athletes and even race horses recover from sports injuries faster with massage.

AT HOME WITH MASSAGE

Touch is so powerful that it can soothe the mind almost as much as the body. The bonus of being able to massage your partner, family or friends at home is that you can treat many of the things for which doctors can only prescribe pills. These include depression, irritability, tension, tiredness, insomnia, stress and bad moods.

Another bonus of doing it in the privacy of your own home is that many people who are too shy or too uncomfortable to have a massage with a stranger, find that they can lie back, relax and enjoy it when it is done by a friend. Not only that, but people of all ages can benefit – babies will fall asleep during the massage on page 115, and grandparents will be fitter for life after the massage on page 25.

(Left) We use touch every day to soothe and comfort both children and adults.

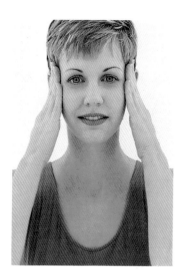

It is easy to learn massage at home. You might not have been taught at school, but the good news is that, unlike mathematics or French, it is easier to pick up at a later stage in life. This is because the first rule of massage is feel rather than think – and as long as it feels good, you are doing it right.

HOW TO MASSAGE

This book has been designed so that you quickly master all the basic tips, tricks and techniques for different massages. Learn the simple hand movements on page 14, read the rules of when not to massage (page 17), study the routine for the chosen ailment and, from then on, improvise.

The main thing is that you must enjoy massage. If you try to balance the book in one hand and turn the pages with oily fingers it will not be much fun. Instead, prop the book up, open on the right page, to remind you of the steps as you go along. Do not be frightened to use the basic strokes, but add your own special touches. Even if you follow one of the routines exactly, repeat the strokes that seem to give the most pleasure – you will soon learn which these are because your 'patient' will grunt, sigh, moan or fall asleep!

Doing the same stroke over and over again is one of the secrets of a really good massage. You do not need to do hundreds of clever thumb contortions to make someone feel good. You can even use the same single, rubbing movement throughout a 30-minute massage and make it feel very different just by varying the

(Right) A soothing massage can be a true gift of love for your partner.

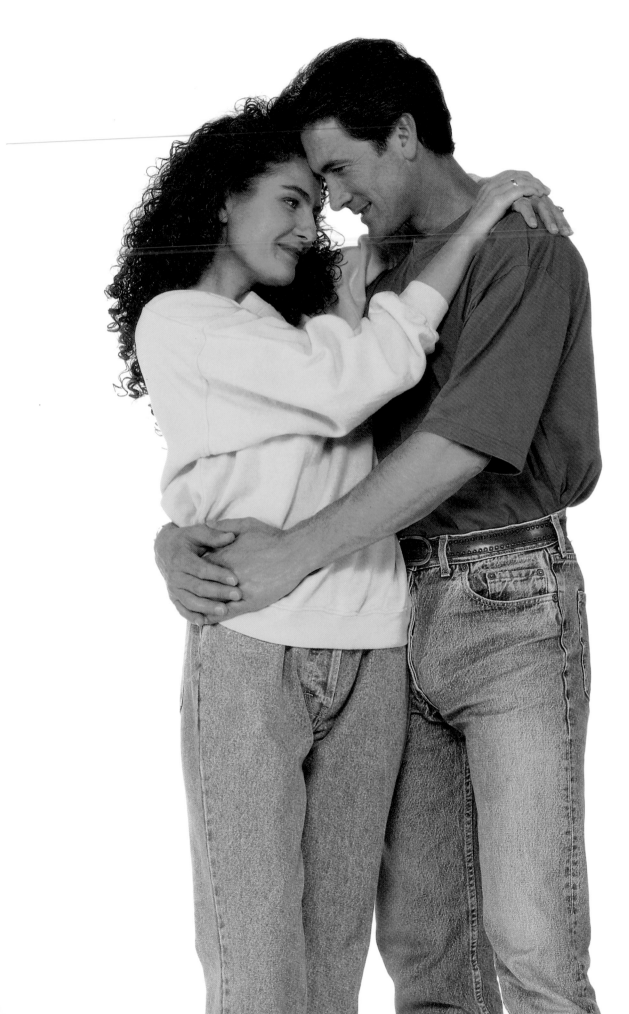

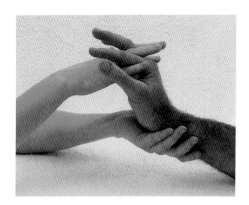

amount of downward pressure, speed and rhythm, changing direction or making long
or short strokes. The more you experiment and follow your instincts,
the more you and the person you are massaging will enjoy it.

As a general rule, soft and slow strokes are soothing, while firm and brisk ones are
invigorating. So you instantly have the power to relax or energize someone just by
altering the speed of a massage. You can do different strokes one after the other in any
order, as long as you keep the same rhythm going during the changeover.

LYING IN COMFORT

The best position to do any massage is the most comfortable one. You need a firm, flat
surface: a futon, a 5-8 cm (2-3 inch) thick foam squab placed on the floor or on a
table top, or a bed big enough for you to kneel or sit on. If the person you are
massaging is lying on his back, a folded towel or pillow behind the nape of the neck
and under the knees will relax the body, especially if he has sore muscles,
a bad back or aching legs. If he is lying on his tummy, a rolled towel
under the collar bone will help relax the neck.

You should wear loose, comfortable clothing and, as you are the one who is doing all
the exercise, something short-sleeved is best or you will get too hot. The room
needs to be very warm, as the body temperature will drop once skin is exposed; it
helps if it is dimly lit and quiet. You will find that some people want to doze off
during a massage, and others unburden themselves by talking non-stop
as they start to relax – either way, you should follow their lead.

(Right) By relaxing the body completely, massage can solve many sleeping problems.

What You Need for Massage

Plenty of spare towels or blankets
and pillows, for warmth
and comfort.

•

A snug, comfortable, well-heated,
cosy room, with dim lighting.

A flat, firm surface to lie on,
with a clean sheet
to protect it from oil.

•

A small, plastic, flip-top bottle
for oil and a basin to warm it in.

•

Peace and quiet.
The rule is, you should only talk if the recipient does.

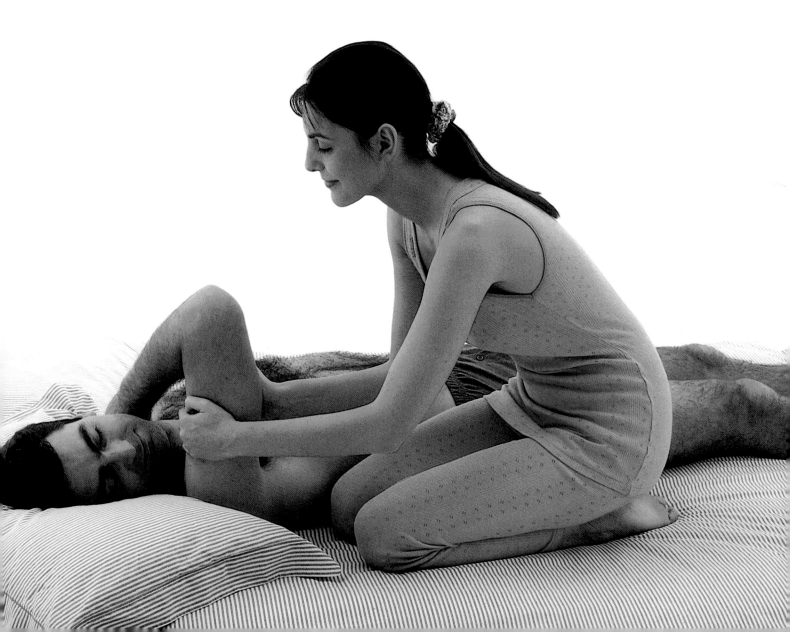

KNOW YOUR STROKES

There are only ten simple massage strokes you need to learn before you can do all 20 of the routines in this book. The easiest way is to practise each one on the top of your thigh so that when you read it in one of the massage steps, you already know what to do.

It also helps you to massage someone else if you know what feels best, so try one of the massages you can do yourself (Massage for Sore Feet, page 99, The Anti-cellulite Massage, page 61, or Beautifying Facial Massage, page 37) and experiment with different speeds, touches and pressures for each stroke.

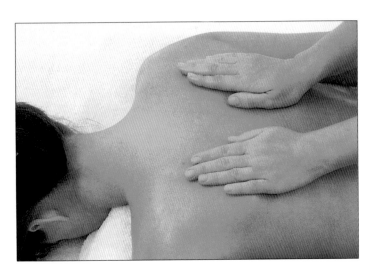

Stroking

This is the simplest movement, with palms down and hands flat (on large areas) or curved (round small areas). You can do it with your fingers only, or you can cat stroke: one hand follows the other and curves so only your fingertips touch at the end of the stroke.

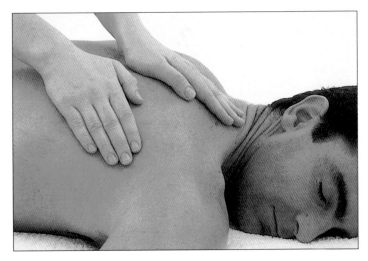

Circling

The hands are in just the same position as for stroking, but they move in circles – one clockwise, the other anti-clockwise. Alternatively, place one hand on the other, palms down, and make a single circle. You can also use both hands, so each completes half of the same circle.

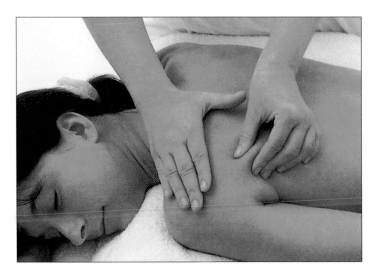

Kneading

Place your hands flat, fingers together with thumbs stretched out wide. Then use your thumbs to push into, squeeze and pinch the flesh up towards the fingers, moving your hands one after the other over the same area of the body.

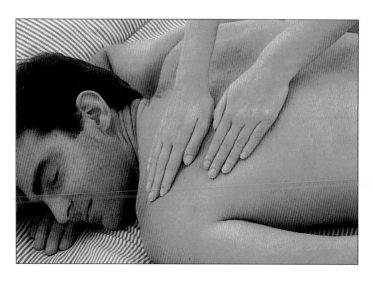

Friction Rub

With palms down and hands flat, move one hand up while the other moves down, in a short, fast sawing movement. You can also do it with the side of your hands, so that you rub with the little finger and the edge of the palm, or with stiff, straight fingers only.

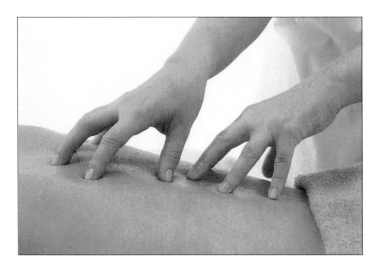

Raking

Imagine your fingertips are the end of a rake – keep them bent at the joints, but stiff. With your fingertips touching the skin, make firm, pulling movements back towards you. Use both hands together or one after the other.

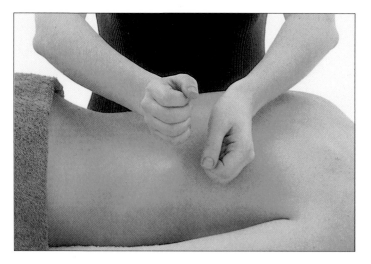

Pummelling

Make your hands into fists and keep your fingers relaxed. Bounce them in a fast drumming movement, one after the other, lightly up and down on the body. You can do it with hands flat, sideways, or palms upwards.

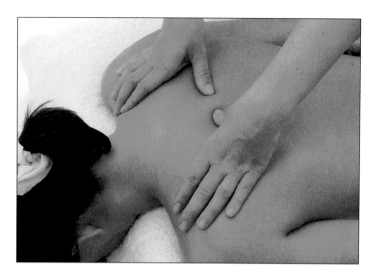

Thumbing

Use the pads and sides of your thumbs to knead into the flesh or stroke deeply. You can also make small, deep circles with thumb tips, or use them to press down, hold, then release over deep muscle tissue (i.e. up the back on either side of the spine).

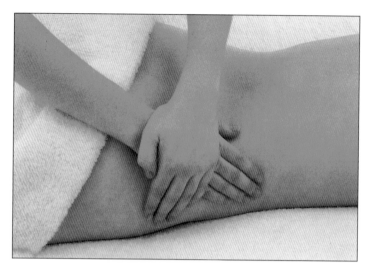

Pressing

You can use this with almost any stroke, to help relax and release muscle tension. For large muscles, place one palm on top of the other, press down for a count of ten, then release. Or press using just the heels of your hands or your index fingers in smaller areas.

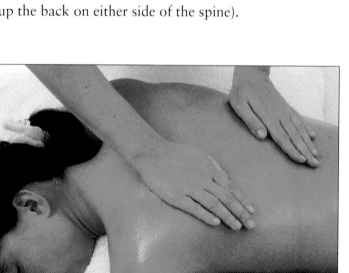

Stretching

This is a downward pressure of hands, palms flat, as you slide them apart in opposite directions to pull and stretch muscles and skin. You can also turn them in opposite directions (i.e. around arms or legs) to twist and wring as you stretch.

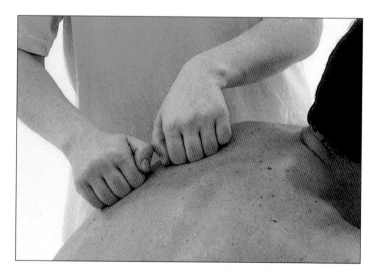

Knuckling

Make your hands into loose fists and place them with fingertips flat on the skin. Roll them forward and turn them right over, so the knuckles push and slide into the skin. You can also do the stroke with the palms of your fists up and just rub your knuckles across the skin.

THE WELL-OILED SKIN

To ensure that your hands slide and slip and warm skin during any massage, you need to cover them with oil. The best types are neither too thin (such as mineral oil), nor too sticky (such as olive oil). Cold-pressed vegetable oils are best, although some, such as coconut and peanut, are rather pungent.

When massaging, keep a small, plastic, flip-top bottle of your chosen oil nearby. Glass bottles easily slip out of oily hands and break, so use plastic if possible. Always warm oils before you apply them by standing the bottle in a basin of hot water for a few minutes.

You need to apply enough oil to make your hands slip, but not slide. Start with a small amount and warm and spread it on the skin, stroking all over with the palms of your hands for several minutes before you do any steps of the actual massage routine. As you spread the oil, feel for any tight muscles, knots or tense areas to come back to later. Add more oil throughout the massage when you need it.

THE DO'S AND DON'TS OF MASSAGE

Massage is one of the safest leisure activities there is, as long as you follow a few basic rules.

- When doing any stroke, never put heavy downward pressure on bony areas or organs (i.e. spine, ribs, shoulders, elbows, knees, abdomen, kidneys).
- When giving a massage, be aware of your own posture so that you do not strain or hurt yourself. Keep your back flat as you bend forward, do not hunch your shoulders, and lengthen your spine and neck.
- If any stroke or movement hurts you or the person you are massaging, stop immediately. Assume that even a wince means that it hurts.
- Do not talk, unless the person you are massaging does. If you have to hold a stroke and count, do not do it aloud.
- Always warm your hands and the oil before you start.

- Always spread oil across the skin with smooth strokes for several minutes before you start massaging.

Best Body Oils

sweet almond

sunflower

safflower

soya

sesame seed

grapeseed

•

Best Facial Oils

peach kernel

apricot

sweet almond

avocado

evening primrose

jojoba

WHEN NOT TO MASSAGE

Although massage really can work miracles, there are occasions when it should not be done. Do not massage someone unless you get a go-ahead from a doctor if they have any of the following conditions:

- Skin infections or any contagious disease.
- Any form of cancer.
- Recent scar tissue or have had recent surgery.
- High temperature or fever.
- Varicose veins, thrombosis or any heart or circulatory problems.
- Epilepsy, asthma or any severe respiratory problems.
- Recurrent or severe back pain, or a long-term injury.
- If the person is ill, frail or there is any doubt whether he should be massaged, check with a doctor first.
- Any form of cancer.

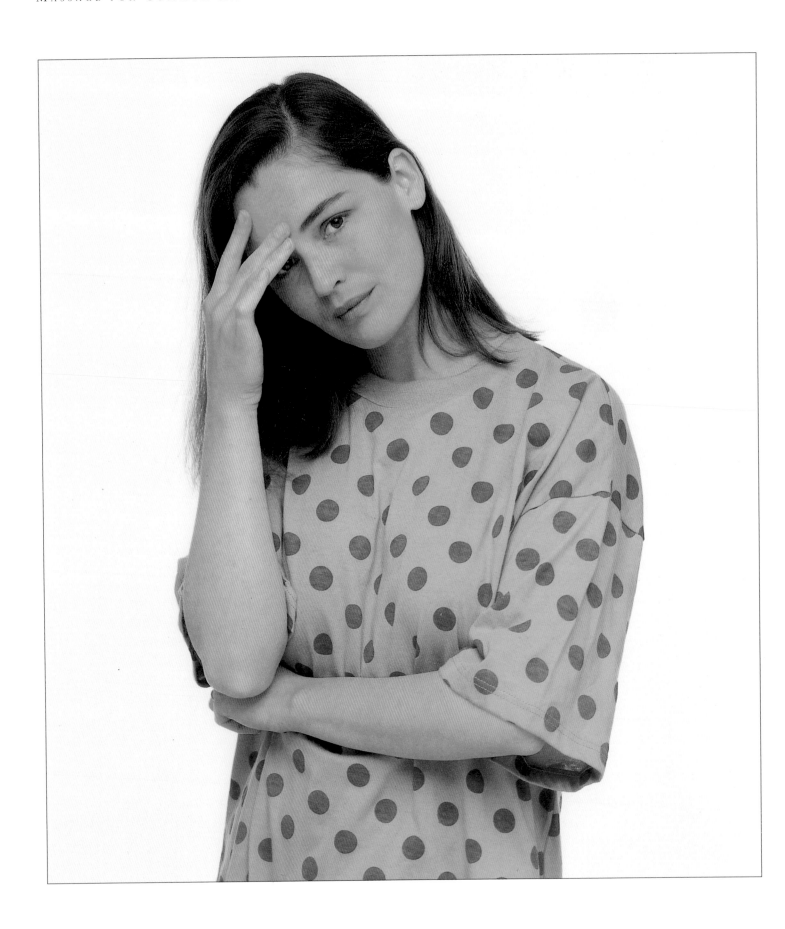

THE RELAXING BODY MASSAGE

It is known that stress is a contributing factor to almost everything that ails modern man. On its simplest level, a little tension leaves you with butterflies in the tummy as the only physical sign. At the other end of the scale, when you suffer from constant, long-term stress and mental anxiety, you can end up with headaches, insomnia, loss of appetite, high blood pressure, nausea, loss of libido, low resistance, even a heart attack.

However, stress in itself is not a bad thing – without it, we would not strive quite so hard or aim quite so high. It is how we react to stress that makes it have a good or bad effect on our bodies. As even the most serious attack of stress can be instantly relieved the second we relax, the best way to react to it is to have a massage.

Massage works by relaxing the muscular tension that builds up to cause more serious symptoms. The hand stroking simply rubs it away. It also relaxes an over-anxious mind by slowing the heartbeat and lowering blood pressure the way yoga, for instance, does. So you feel better both physically and mentally in one go.

As there is less and less time in life for leisure, hobbies and sports, massage is even more important as a way to relax – it is quick, simple and needs no fancy equipment or membership fees. Also, it is just about impossible to injure yourself. If you have regular relaxing massages, you will never be tense and will be healthier and happier throughout your life.

HOW TO DO A RELAXING BODY MASSAGE

To do a full body massage properly takes an hour, but this one can be done in 30 minutes since it concentrates only on the areas where tension hits worse. It uses a series of presses, stretches and deep strokes, as these are the best instant tension busters. However, the more you repeat strokes the better it feels, so extend it as much as time allows.

The massage is meant to relax, so help as much as possible. Keep the room dimly lit, warm and quiet and use plenty of pillows, blankets and oil.

(Left) Through a variety of aches and pains, your body will alert you to tension.

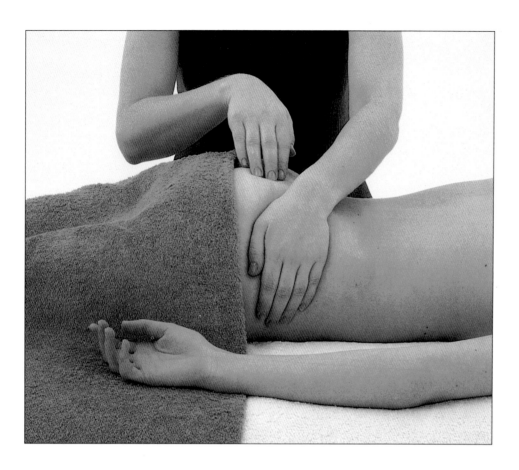

1 ◄ For steps one, two and three, the person being massaged should lie face down, and for steps four onwards, she should lie face up. Start at the feet, placing your hands, palms down, for a firm, slow full body stroke up the calves, thighs, over the buttocks, up each side of the back to the top of the shoulders, then stroking down the arms to the palms of the hands. Repeat. Next make firm circular strokes in unison up the legs, with your left hand anti-clockwise and right hand clockwise. Cover the lower body with blankets. Move up to the waist and do side stroking. Tuck your fingers down under the hip and pull one hand after the other upwards in a smooth, flowing motion. Take several minutes to work up to the top of the waist, then repeat on the other side.

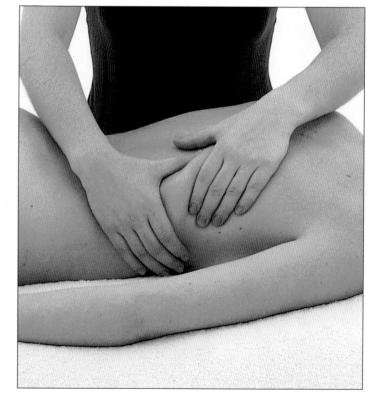

2 ▶ First stretch the back: place both hands, palms down, over the spine in the middle of the back and pull your hands in opposite directions so that one ends on the tailbone and the other at the nape of the neck. Concentrate on stretching the body and not pressing down. Repeat. Then spend a long time kneading all over the back, pinching and squeezing the flesh between thumb and fingers of both hands, from the buttocks to shoulder tops, avoiding bony areas.

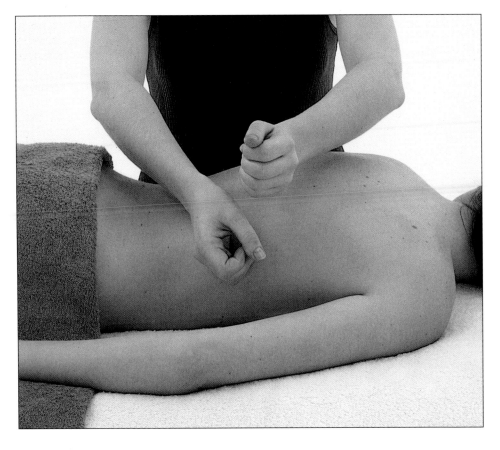

3 ◀ Pummel the middle and upper back, using the base of loose fists for several minutes. Avoid kidneys and spine. The person being massaged should now turn face up. Cover the upper body. Place the palms over the top of each foot, fingers pointing upwards, and stroke firmly several times from ankle to knee. Repeat the stroke from the upper knee to thigh top, using a firmer pressure. Then place the thumbs on one side of the thigh, fingers on the other and knead. Do a fast friction rub all over the thigh, then repeat on the other thigh.

4 ▼ Repeat the full body stroke from step one, but on the front. This time end by pressing the heels of your hands for a count of ten where the arms join the chest. Push gently for a count of five over biceps, elbow creases, wrists and palms. Then, with her palms down, hold one of her forearms with one hand. Place the other hand over the wrist, then push up, pressing lightly, to the shoulder. Repeat several times on both arms.

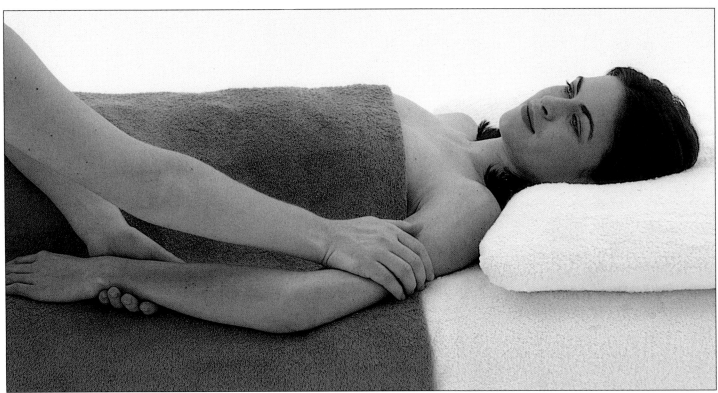

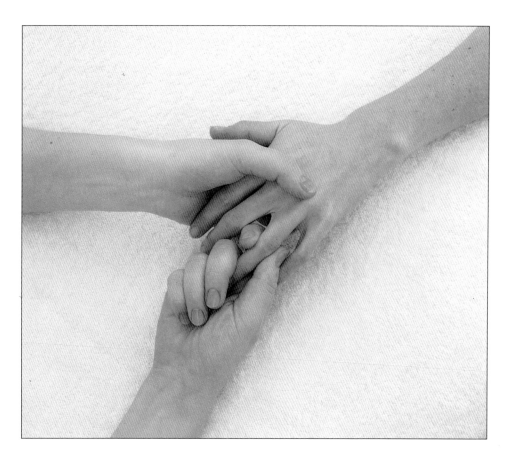

5 ◀ Cover the body to keep it warm. Pick up one hand of the person being massaged and, supporting it with your left palm under the wrist, gently push her fingers up with the palm of your right hand to stretch the hand backwards. Hold for a count of six, then relax. Turn her hand palm up and place it in the palm of your right hand, using your straight fingers to support it as you make firm strokes with your thumb from her wrist to her fingers. Finish by grasping each finger between your thumb and index finger as you pull from the base to the tip, twisting round in a corkscrew motion. Repeat all of the strokes on the other hand.

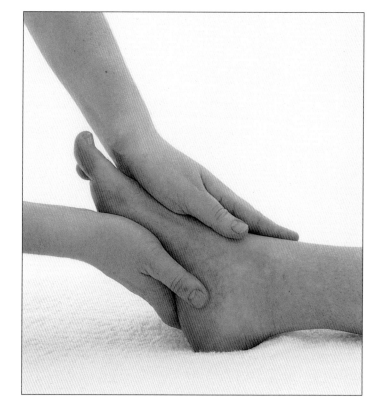

6 ▶ Now work on the feet. First massage the sole of the left foot with your thumbs, supporting the foot with your fingers wrapped round the instep. Make firm strokes (under the arch and toes) and circles (from heels up to toes) all over the sole of the foot. Then sandwich the foot between the palms of your hands at the ankle and pull firmly as you draw your hands back off the tips of the toes. Repeat this pull several times in a smooth, flowing stroke. Hold each toe between your thumb and index finger and twist round as you pull from the base to the tip. Repeat all strokes on the other foot.

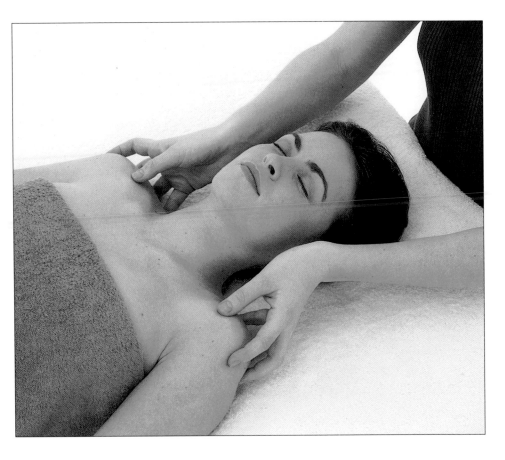

7 ◀ Cover the whole body and move up to stand at the head. Place one hand, palm up, under the back between the shoulder blades and draw it firmly up the neck to the base of the skull, keeping your fingers outstretched and slightly arching the neck. Repeat using the other hand and continue as a flowing stroke. Then, with palms flat, stroke from the top of the arm up the side of the neck, one hand following the other. Repeat on the other side. With stiff, bent fingers, rake the same area from arm to neck, making firm, fast strokes with both hands working together, one on each shoulder.

8 ▶ Placing your fingers together, use palms and fingers to 'cat' stroke up the sides of the neck. 'Cat' stroke means stroking with your fingers curved in a convex direction. Place palms down over each shoulder top and push down. Hold for a count of 15, then relax. Use the sides of your thumbs to make slow circles in a clockwise direction over each temple for two minutes. Then lightly press your fingertips over the eyes for a count of 20. Use the tips of both index fingers, one after the other, to do the gentlest stroke up between the eyebrows for two minutes. Then use the palms of your hands, one after the other, to do a firm stroke from brows to crown. With stiff fingers, press into the scalp and make small circles with the fingertips all over the head. Place your left hand, palm up, under the nape of the neck across the skull and your right hand, palm down, on the forehead. Press in firmly with both hands for a count of ten. Relax and repeat.

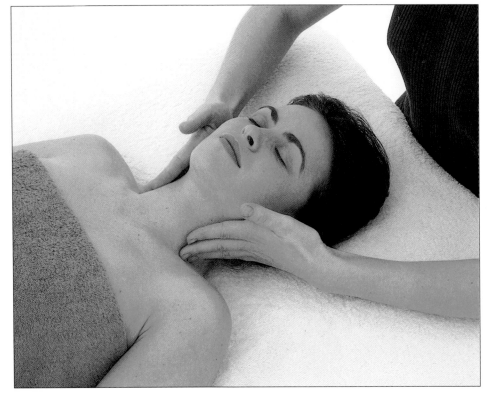

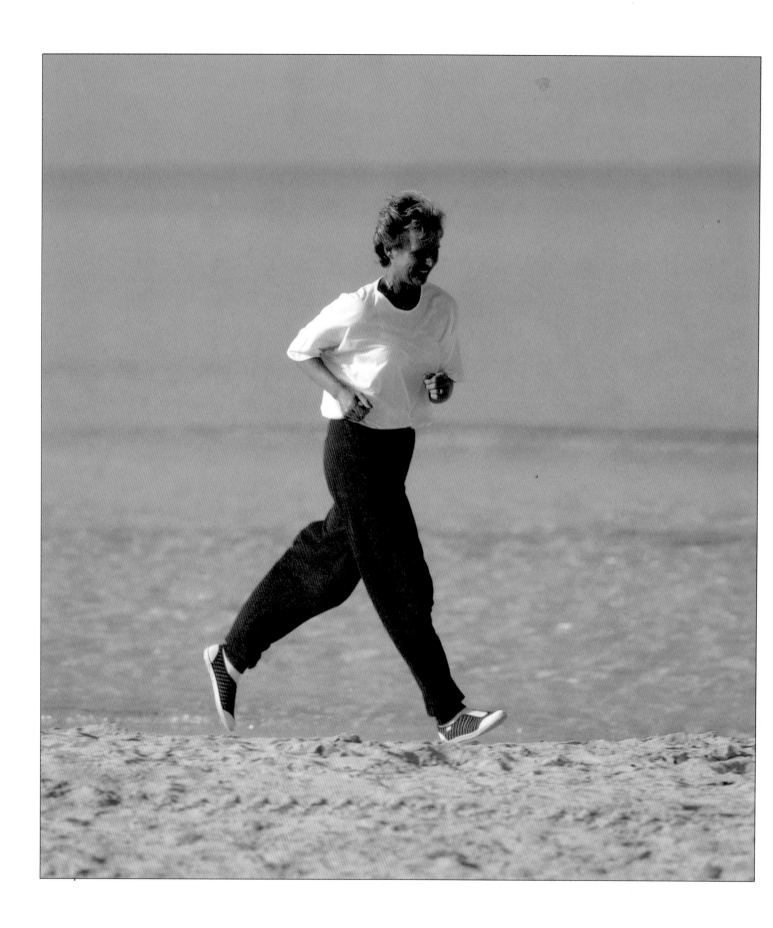

THE FIT FOR LIFE MASSAGE

This decade has seen a new approach to ageing and now most of us expect to look and feel younger than our parents did as we grow older. It is not just wishful thinking – research shows that from the age of 25 onwards, more than half of 'ageing' is not ageing at all. It is the physical signs of a life spent eating too much and exercising too little. The most obvious signs of ageing – middle-aged spread, stiff joints, stooped shoulders, and loss of chest, back and hip mobility – are not only preventable but, in many instances, are reversible.

Experts now say that ten to 15 minutes gentle daily exercise throughout your life will delay body ageing by ten to 20 years. To help keep you moving, this massage has been devised to stretch and rub the muscles that tend to seize up quickest, so your body is as supple, lithe and flexible as possible. As it should be done every day of your life, it is simple (two rubs, six stretches) and speedy (ten minutes from start to finish), so that you can never say you are too busy to do it.

It is never too late or too early to begin. The fit for life massage is perfect to do on children, who like the vigorous strokes and get bored if they have to lie still for more than a few minutes. It is equally good for someone over 70, who may not be comfortable with a slow, hands-on massage or supple enough to do what they think of as 'proper' exercise alone.

HOW TO DO THE FIT FOR LIFE MASSAGE

The first two steps, an all-over friction rub and light pummel, help boost the circulation, warm muscles and relax an inflexible body. The six stretches that follow help increase suppleness and flexibility in the areas that seize up soonest in an ageing body.

The massage may be done with oil and wearing only underwear or towels, or without oil and wearing loose, comfortable clothes. It is best done on the floor or a very firm, low bed so that the body is supported for the stretches. If you are short of time, you can forego the final friction rub in step eight.

(Left) Suppleness is the key to being fit for life: keep moving to stay younger, longer.

1 Steps one to four should be done with the person being massaged lying face down. Start with a circulation-boosting, all-over friction rub. Work in an upwards direction, from feet to legs, buttocks, back, then hands and arms. Do a fast, sawing back and forwards motion, changing the stroke by using palms flat down, sides of hands only, heels of hands only, or stiff fingertips.

2 Next do a pummelling stroke, working in an upwards direction from the soles of feet, calves, thighs, buttocks, upper back and shoulders. Bounce your hands off the skin, firmly on large dense muscles and with a lighter flick on bony or sensitive parts. Vary the stroke by using your flat fists, the backs of your knuckles, flicking with loose fingers, or using the base of your fists like hammers.

3 ▼ Cross the legs of the person being massaged at the ankle and slowly take both feet up, then bend them gently down towards the buttocks. Stop as soon as you feel resistance, and hold the stretch for a count of 15 before releasing and dropping the feet back to the floor. Repeat the stretch twice more, but never go so far that it causes discomfort.

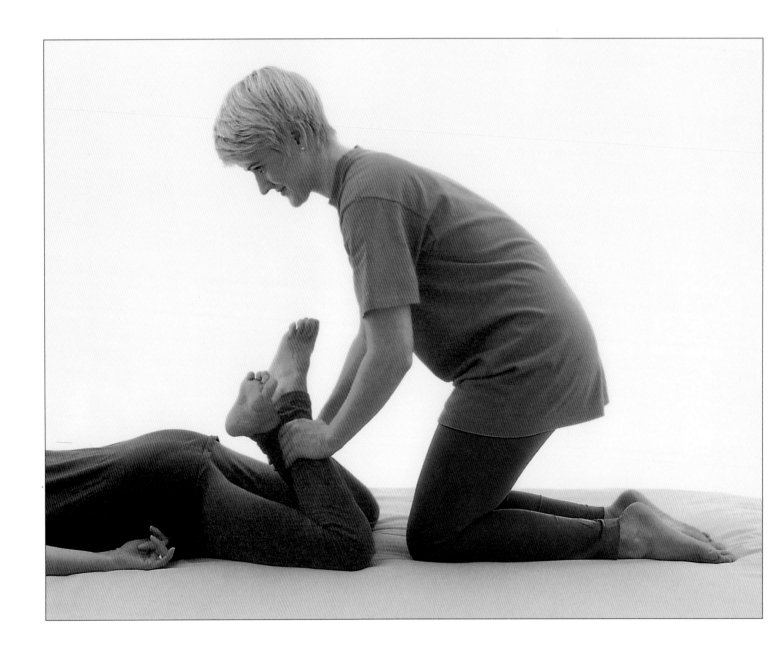

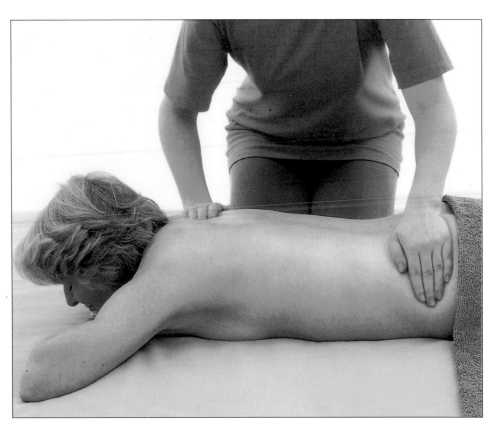

4 ◀ Lightly place your hands, palms down, in the middle of the back. Then do a cross-stretch by sliding one hand to the hip as the other goes to the opposite shoulder – the skin should stretch between your hands while you hold for a count of ten. Relax, then repeat on the other shoulder and hip. From the same start position, do another stretch the length of the back, so that one hand ends at the neck and the other on the tailbone. Repeat.

5 ▼ The person being massaged should turn over so she is lying face up, with her legs straight out. Cross her legs at the ankle and gently raise the feet so that the knees bend up to the chest. Stop as soon as you meet resistance, and hold the stretch for a count of 15 before releasing and lowering the feet back to the floor. Repeat the stretch twice more.

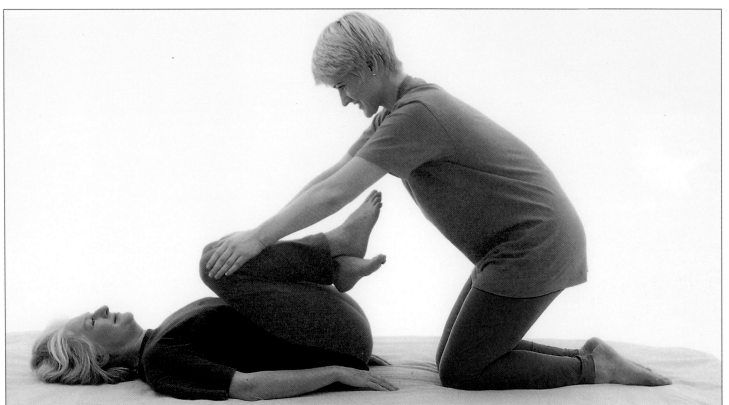

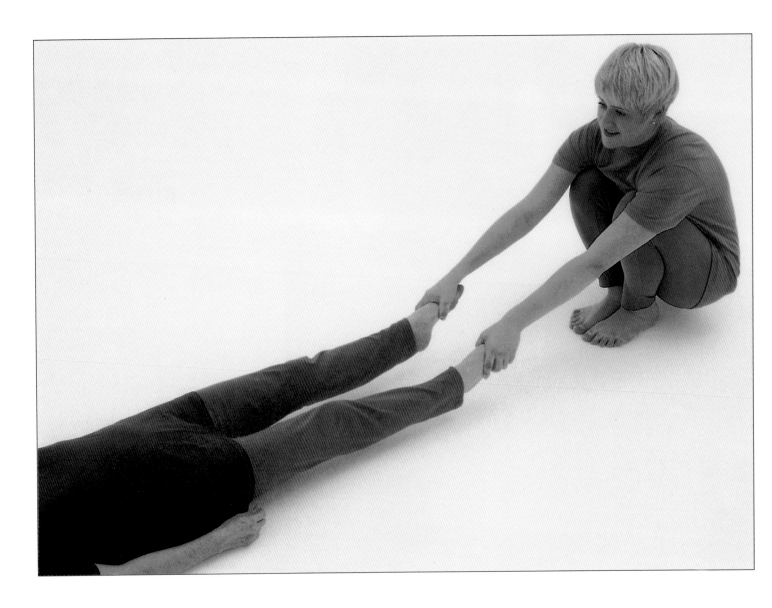

6 ▲ While the person being massaged is lying straight out, stand at her feet and grasp firmly around the top of each foot and toes. Crouch down and extend your arms to lean back and gently pull her legs away from her body. Hold the stretch for a count of 15 before releasing. Then repeat once.

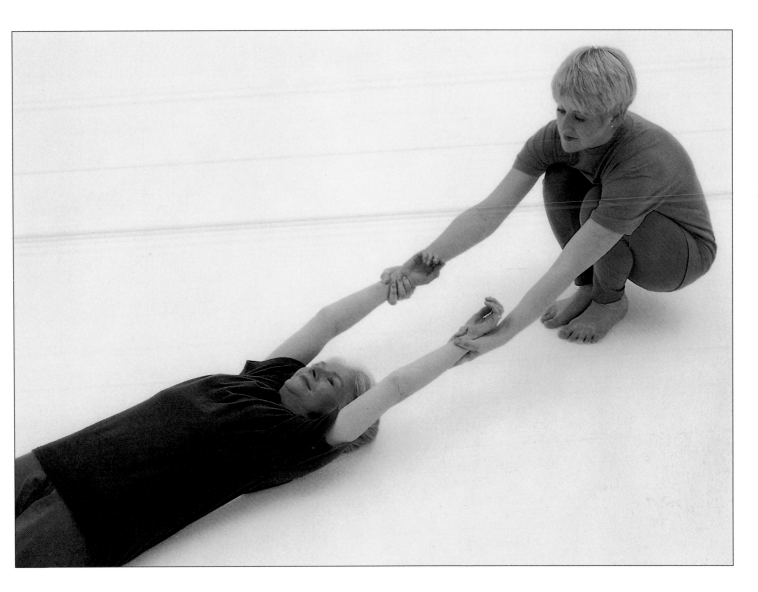

7 ▲ Stand at her head and hold both her hands by grasping firmly around the wrists and forearms. Crouch down and extend your arms, keeping her arms raised at a 45° angle throughout, and lean back to pull her arms gently away from her body. Hold for a count of 15, relax, then repeat.

8 ▶ Slide the fingers of each hand under the nape of her neck and interlock them across the vertebrae so that your palms are flat. *Gently* lift up to stretch and arch the neck, keeping the top of the head on the floor for support. Hold the stretch for a count of ten, then relax. Finish off by repeating step one again, doing the feet, legs, thighs, hands and arms and always working in an upwards direction.

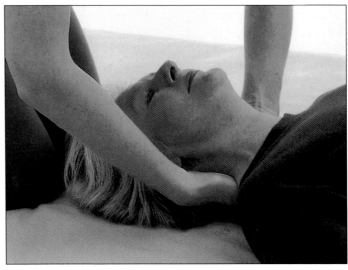

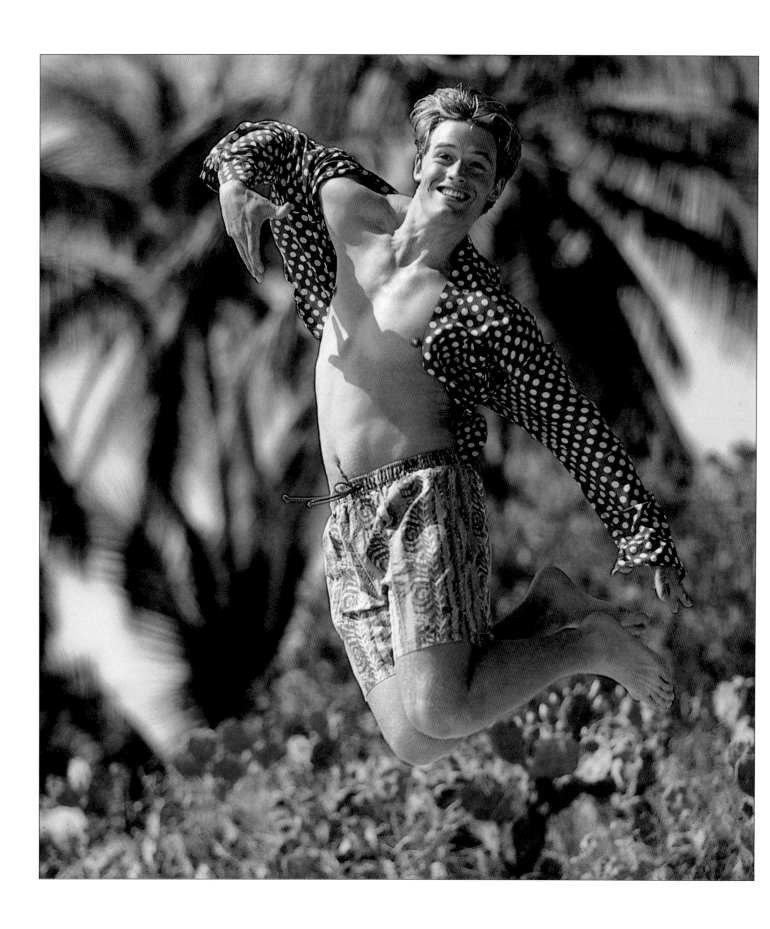

THE ENERGIZING BODY MASSAGE

These days life is such a rat race that many of us feel like little rodents spinning round on their wheels – always racing to the next hurdle, but never quite getting there. If you put in an eight-hour day at work, followed by two hours with the children and three hours trying to organize everything that needs to be done, it is often absolutely exhausting. The feeling of low energy is not caused by physical activity so much as by mental anxiety.

When we encounter the hundreds of things every day and all day that make us tense, our blood pressure automatically rises and energy reserves fall. This is the worst kind of tiredness. If you are physically exhausted, you fall asleep, but if you are mentally exhausted, you keep going – without your sense of humour and without any patience or pleasure in what you are doing.

Massage really can help energize anyone who is overtired by rubbing away the physical signs of stress and releasing tension from muscles. The firmer, faster strokes invigorate both mind and body in the same way that waking up to a cold shower will.

HOW TO DO AN ENERGIZING BODY MASSAGE

Although, like all massages, this one is more pleasurable done on bare skin, it is effective done through clothing. Consequently, it is ideal for those times when you get home exhausted and need an energy-boost before you go out again.

The best positions for the person being massaged are sitting sideways on a straight-backed chair and bent forward onto a pillow on a desk or table top in front, or sitting facing the back of a chair and leaning forwards onto a pillow propped against the chair back. If you are doing it on bare skin, use plenty of oil for the friction or pummelling strokes to stop your hands dragging.

The main massage movements are done from the waist to head, but you can make it more invigorating by doing the optional extra energizing body shakes described in the box at the end of step eight – and you can also do them alone, just to wake yourself up, clear your head or increase energy at any time during a busy day.

(Left) The energizing massage will leave you raring to go rather than ready for bed.

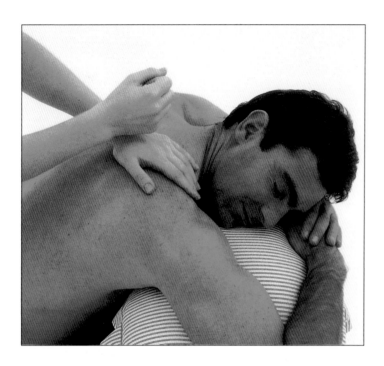

1 ◄ With the person being massaged leaning forward onto a pillow, pummel all over the upper back, avoiding the spine. Place one hand, palm down and flat, make a firm fist with the other hand and bounce it up and down on top of the flat hand, moving all over the top of the back for several minutes. This stroke is meant to simply vibrate the muscles rather than be a forceful punch.

2 ► Then make a light 'pinky' finger slap all over the same area. This is a quick up-and-down stroke, as if you are shaking water off your fingers. Use the whole of the little finger and just the tips of the middle and ring fingers to make contact with the back, keeping them floppy and loose. One hand should follow the other, in a light, relaxed flick.

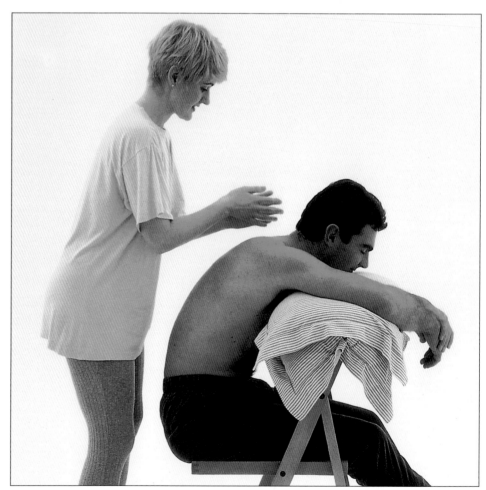

3 ▶ Knead the muscles across the tops of the shoulders by squeezing the flesh between your thumbs and fingers for several minutes. Then place your forearms on the shoulders, keeping your hands relaxed and your fingers hanging down loosely. Gently lean down, using your bodyweight to press the muscle across the shoulder top in a downward stretch. Only be as firm as is comfortable, hold the stretch for a count of ten, then relax. Holding the arm tops, gently push the shoulders forward, hold, then release and pull them back to stretch.

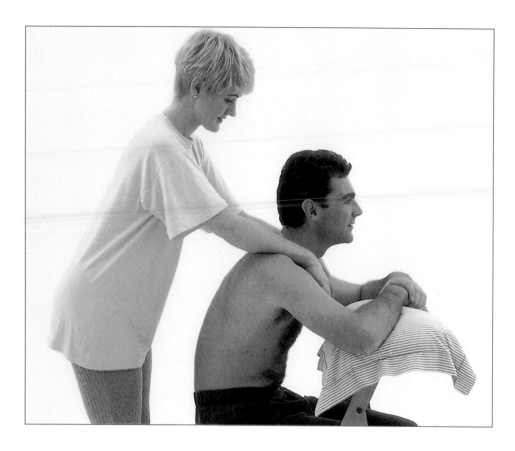

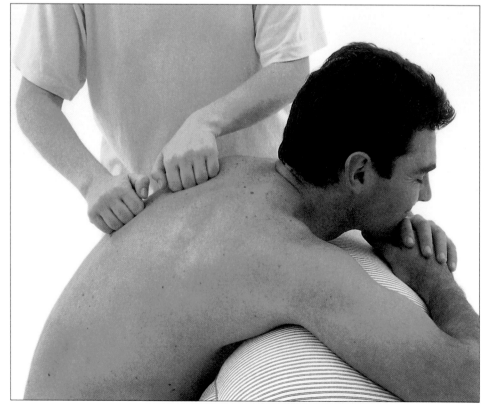

4 ◀ Roll your knuckles down one side of the spine from the nape of the neck to the buttock. Start 5 cm (2 inches) away from the spine and roll across the long muscles that run parallel to the vertebrae. Make a firm fist, then press the flat part of the fingertips down into the muscle as you roll your hand forward, pressing down through the finger joints and knuckles throughout the roll. Roll one hand after the other continuously, gradually working down the back. Then repeat on the other side.

5 ▶ Place flat, firm hands, palms down, on the lower back on either side of the spine, about 5 cm (2 inches) away from it. Slide one hand up as one goes down in a slow, deep, firm stroke so that the skin is being stretched and pulled in opposite directions. Gradually work from the lower back up to the shoulder tops.

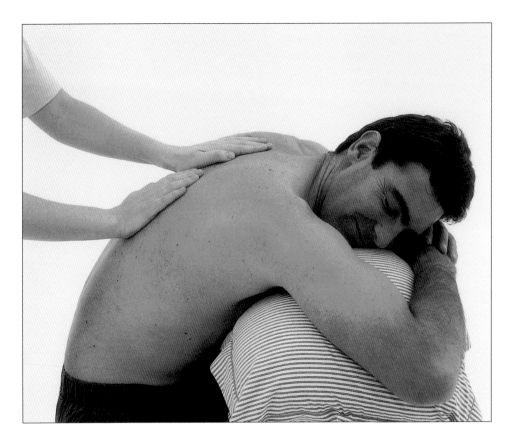

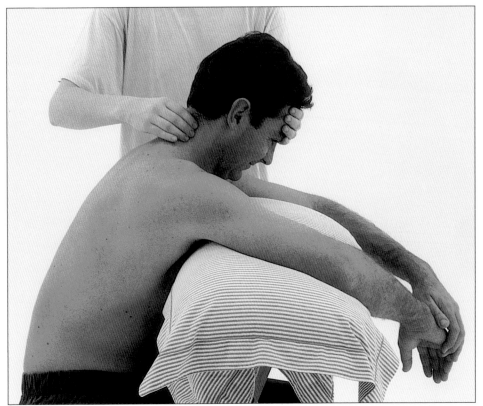

6 ◀ Place the palm of your left hand on the forehead to support the head as the person being massaged bends forward. Place your thumb and fingers on either side of the vertebrae and knead from the nape of the neck up to the skull bone. Then, using thumbs only, make small circles over the same area.

7 ▼ Next, with stiff, straight fingers, rake and gently scrub all over the scalp as if shampooing the hair, from the hairline up to the crown. Finish off with long, smooth stiff-finger strokes all over the head. Then use flat loose fingers to slap and tap the head lightly, in a fast up-and-down movement.

8 Using the little fingers and sides of the hands, do a light finger chop across the shoulder tops. Keep your fingers relaxed and bounce them lightly up and down in a flicking motion, with both hands working together on the same side of the neck. Keep the rhythm going for several minutes on each side.

EXTRA ENERGIZING BODY SHAKES

1 Sitting in a chair, turn from the waist and look back as far as you can over one shoulder, hold for a count of six, then look over the other. Repeat.

2 Keeping arms straight, raise one shoulder up as the other goes down, and repeat rapidly 20 times.

3 Press down into the seat of the chair with your palms, then with bent knees, lift up one heel off the floor, followed by the other, as if running on the spot.

4 With relaxed, loose arms, shake your hands vigorously as if flicking water from them. Repeat with them above your head.

5 With your shoulders straight, shake your head as if flicking water from your hair.

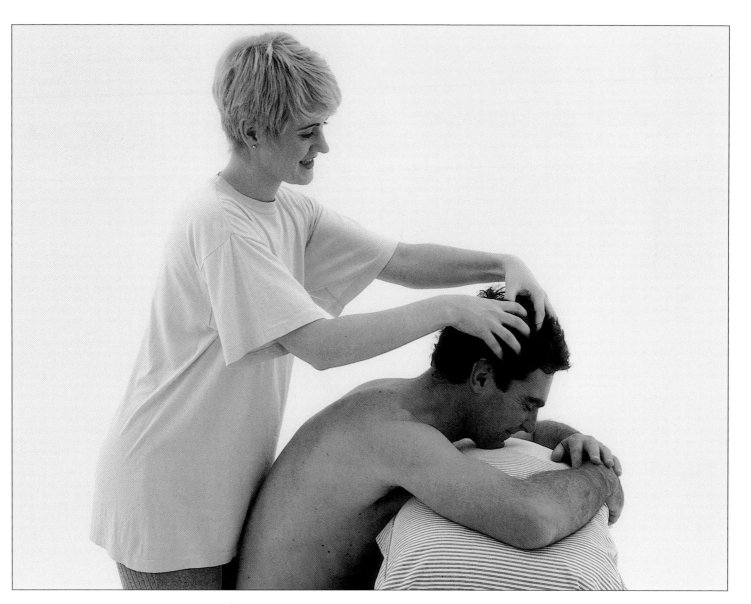

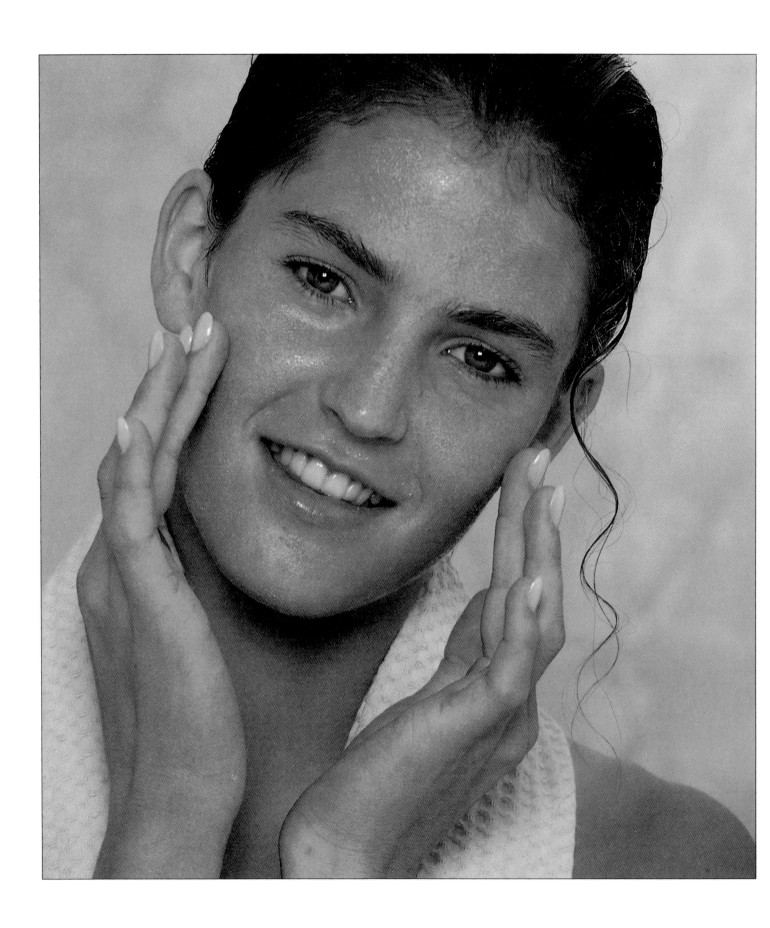

BEAUTIFYING FACIAL MASSAGE

The good news is that a face massage is one of the best beauty treatments you can give yourself. The bad news is that, unfortunately, it does not exercise the muscles, stop the skin sagging, prevent wrinkles or act as a natural facelift. Over 80 per cent of wrinkles are caused by sun damage, the rest are hereditary; both are impossible to wipe away with the stroke of a hand. The best two weapons against premature wrinkling are protecting skin from the sun and making sure it is always well moisturized.

However, although massage cannot make you look younger, it can definitely make you look good for your age. As you massage in creams or oils, the warmth of your hand and the rubbing action ensure that they are better absorbed by the surface skin. This, in turn, means that skin is better moisturized, plumper, softer, has that dewy youthful look and is well protected from the environment.

Massage also releases all the tiny, taut, facial expression muscles so that your complexion immediately looks smoother, more relaxed and less wrinkled. This is the instant beautifying effect that makes you look as serene as the Mona Lisa, even after stressful days and sleepless nights.

HOW TO MASSAGE THE FACE

This is a self-massage, so it is an ideal way for you to apply your daily moisturizer, morning or night. To give your fingers enough slip, you will need more moisturizer than usual but you will find it is quickly and thoroughly absorbed.

Alternatively, massage in a fine facial oil, such as peach kernel, apricot kernel, sweet almond, avocado or wheatgerm. These will not leave a shiny, greasy finish to the skin and are excellent moisturizers – they seal the surface so effectively that they keep more natural moisture in the skin than most cosmetic face creams.

Do the massage sitting in front of a mirror until you are familiar with the movements. Do all strokes with a gentle, light hand – and do step six in private, unless you want to be laughed at!

(Left) A facial massage ensures that your daily moisturizer is absorbed completely.

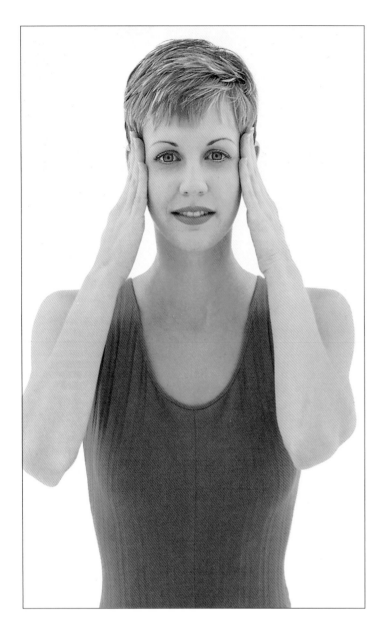

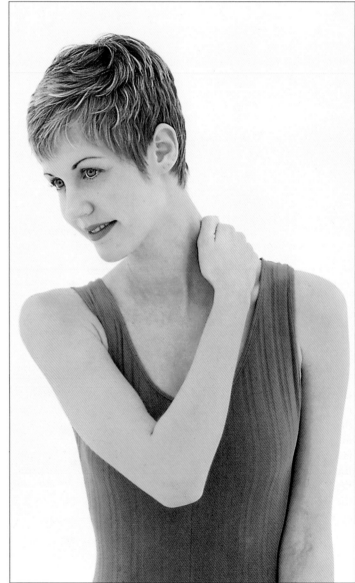

2 ▼ Place your right hand, palm down, on your left shoulder and pull along the shoulder up the neck to the ear, using the whole of the hand for the stroke. This should be a strong, slow, continuous movement to stretch the large shoulder muscles – bending your head slightly to the right will help increase the stretch. To help your right arm make a firm stroke, rest your left arm flat on the table and use it to support your right arm. Repeat several times, then swap sides and use your left hand on your right shoulder.

1 ▲ Start with a long, slow, heart-shaped stroke around the whole face. Place your fingertips on the middle of the chin, then turn them as you run the palms of each hand out along the jaw bone, up over the cheekbones, pushing into the temples and across the top of each eyebrow so that your fingertips meet on the bridge of the nose. Gently press into the eyes for a count of ten, relax and repeat the entire stroke several times. Finish off by firmly stroking five times, one palm after the other, from brows up to the hairline.

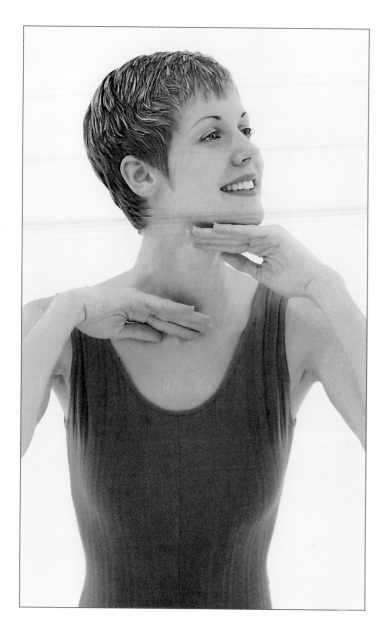

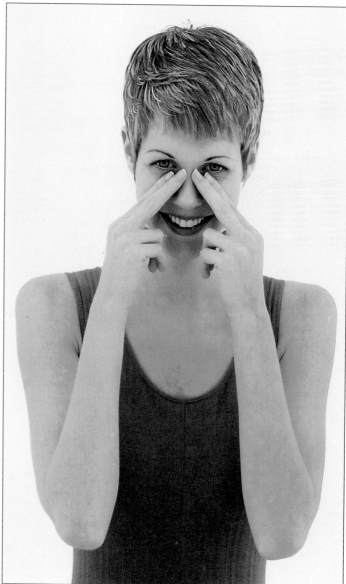

4 ▼ Place your two index fingers on either side of the bridge of the nose. Run them lightly down the length of the nose, around the nostrils and press into the middle of the top lip. Repeat several times. Then place the first two fingers of one hand in the centre of your forehead, run them firmly down the bridge of the nose, open them wide to go around the nostrils and meet again in the middle of the top lip. Finish off by using the same two fingers of each hand firmly to stroke from the bridge of the nose up to the forehead. Repeat.

3 ▲ Place your fingertips, palm up, on the side of your neck level with the collar bone. Pull one hand up after the other in a smooth, flowing, rhythmic movement from the neck up to the jaw, working across and back from ear to ear for several minutes. Then place the backs of both index fingers under your jaw, with nails touching below the chin. Lightly pat so that one finger follows the other, in an upward flicking motion, across the jawline from side to side. Then drop the head back and point the chin up to stretch the neck for a count of five.

5 ▷ Using the middle two fingers, stroke firmly along the line of each eyebrow from inner to outer corner several times. Then lightly place a thumb over each inner eye corner, press gently in, hold for a count of four, relax and repeat, following the contours of the eye socket under the brow to the outer eye. Repeat from outer to inner corner under the eye, using index fingers rather than thumbs. Finish off by gently pressing in over the tear ducts, so that you have made a complete circle of little presses right around each eye.

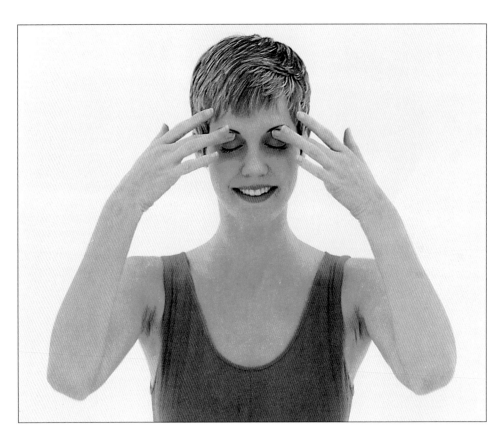

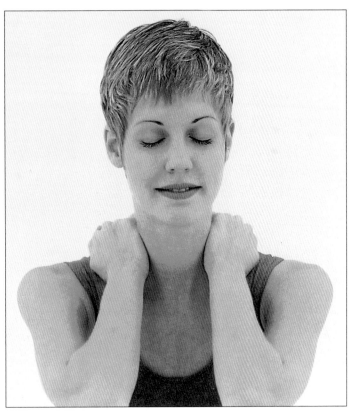

6 ◁ Leaning forwards on your elbows, place the palm of each hand on either side of the neck. Keeping your head and chin dropped forwards throughout, press in deeply with your fingertips and make small circles all across the shoulder muscles. Then in the same position, point the chin up, drop the head back, and pinch, press, squeeze and knead the shoulder muscles. Finally, press in firmly with your hands in the same position while you make exaggerated 'A, E, I, O, U' vowel sounds out loud. Do these repeatedly and quickly to relax the jaw and neck.

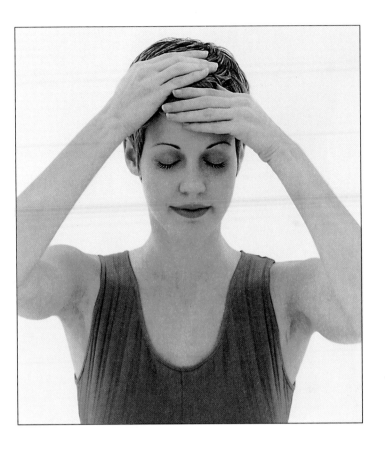

7 ◀ Repeat step one, doing a full-face, heart-shaped stroke from chin up over cheeks to the temples. This time, when you reach the brows, finish the stroke by moving palms up the forehead into the hair four or five times quite firmly. Then place the first two fingers of each hand over each temple and press firmly inwards. Move the fingers in slow circles without releasing the pressure, so that the skin is stretched with the circular movement. Finish off by pressing firmly into the temples for a count of ten, then relax.

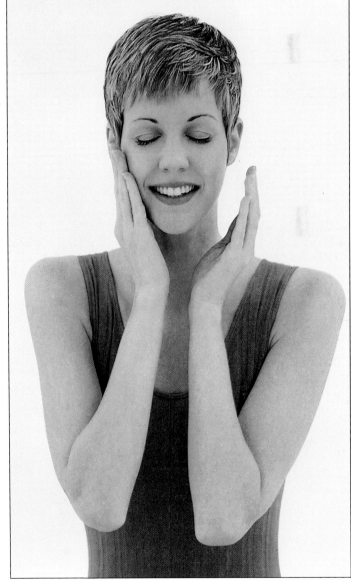

8 ▶ Keeping the fingers of one hand stiff, place it palm down so that your fingertips rest between the brows. Make figure-of-eight shapes by stroking out over the left brow, down and under the left eye, up over the nose, out over the right brow and under the right eye. Keep the stroke flowing and repeat several times. Then place both hands, palms flat, over the face and lightly pat rapidly up and down all over. Finish off by placing the hands, palms down, parallel with the nose and pressing into the face for a count of ten, hold, then relax.

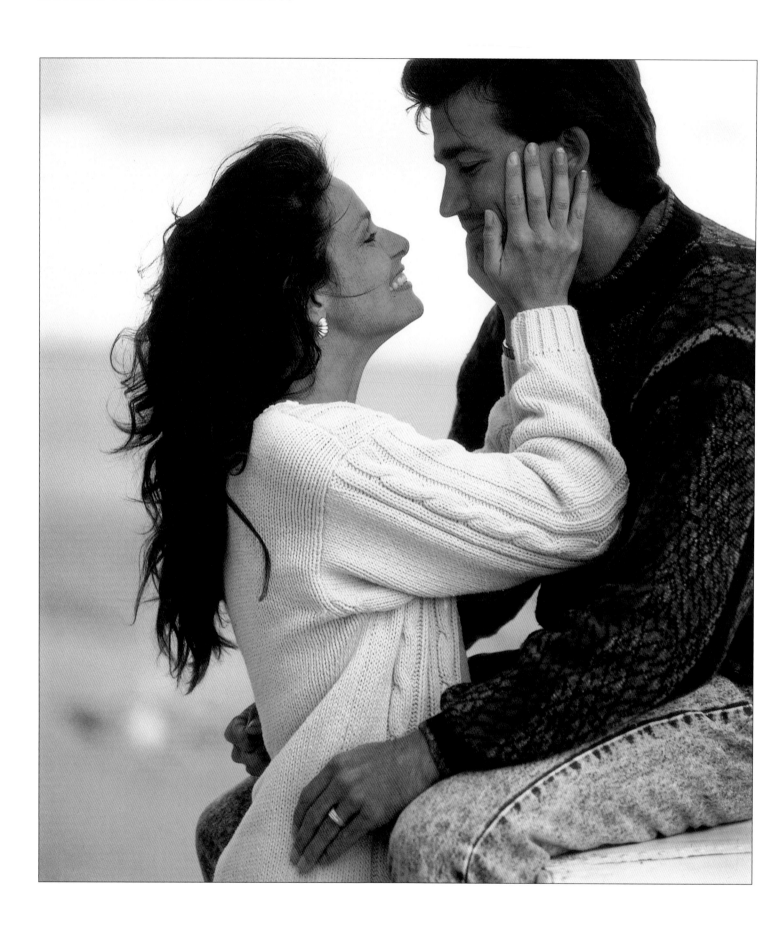

THE CIRCULATION-BOOSTING MASSAGE

＊

This is a massage for arms and legs and feet and hands only. If you have ever suffered from the mid-winter big chill, you will know why. When you get into bed and your partner screams 'Don't touch me', when you put your feet on a hot water bottle and it goes cold, or when your hands are numb even though you have just stoked the fire, you know you have a problem.

The problem is slow circulation and it affects the unlucky all year round. Even at the height of summer, there are some of us who turn over in the night and unwittingly put two blocks of ice in the middle of a loved one's back. However, this massage is not just for the cold-handed, warm-hearted types.

Boosting the circulation is a way of making the whole body healthier. First it stimulates blood flow, so that wastes are swept away and fresh oxygenated blood rushes to every body cell. Then it brings a warm, rosy glow to the skin, so that you look healthy and happy. And finally, it wakes you up, makes you tingle with energy and puts a skip back in your step.

So this massage is equally wonderful, whether you plan to be warmly tucked up in bed or want to have the energy to go out and dance after a long, hard day. It uses lots of fast, firm friction rubs to warm the body and stir up the blood, mixed with firm, slow pushing strokes to make sure that the blood flows rapidly back to the heart. It is also quick to do, easy to master and very beneficial.

HOW TO DO A CIRCULATION-BOOSTING MASSAGE

When doing friction strokes, always keep the movements short and fast, so that one hand moves up and works against the other which is moving down. You need lots of extra oil as the rapid rubbing and heat drives it into skin. Hands can lose slip and drag on the body very quickly.

As it is important to catch all the body heat being generated, have lots of towels or blankets handy to wrap over the parts of the body that you are not working on. The best position is for the person being massaged to lie on the floor or a firm, low bed, and for you to kneel beside her. For steps one to five, she should lie face up, and for steps six to eight, she should lie face down.

(Left) Good circulation brings renewed energy as well as warmer hands and feet!

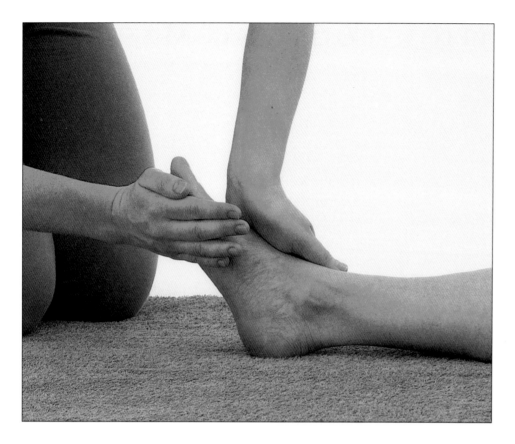

1 ◄ Do steps one to three on the right leg, then repeat all steps on the left leg. Sandwich the foot between the palms of your hands and do a fast, firm friction rub, so one hand moves forward as the other moves back. After several minutes, change to stroking the foot from toes up to ankle, still with one hand on the top and the other on the sole of the foot.

2 ► Raise the right leg and support it by placing your right hand around the back of the ankle. Place your left hand palm down, thumb to front and fingers around the back, and push it firmly up the leg from ankle to knee. Repeat and after the sixth stroke, swap hands so that the right one slides up the other side from ankle to knee for six strokes. Swap and repeat twice more.

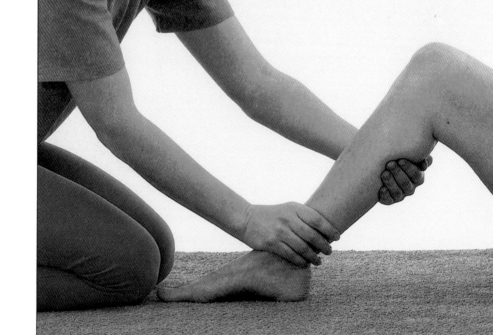

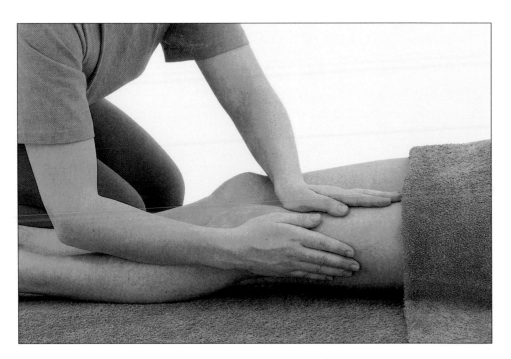

3 ◄ Kneeling by the knees of the person being massaged, place both hands, palms down, on her right thigh. Keeping hands flat, do a fast, firm friction rub all over from knee up to the thigh top for several minutes. Then do some slow, deep, firm strokes in the same area, with fingers relaxed and curved so that you use the heel of your hand. Now repeat steps one to three on the left leg.

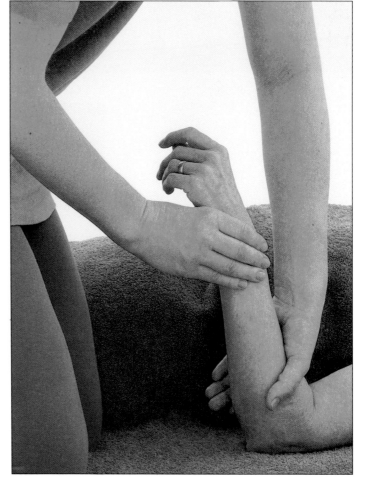

4 ▷ Kneel by the waist of the person being massaged and pick up her left arm, bending it at the elbow. With palms down, hold her wrist so that your thumb is over her pulse and your fingers are wrapped around the forearm. Slide the other hand down towards the elbow, using light finger/thumb pressure. As it reaches the bottom, take it back to the start to hold the wrist while sliding your other hand down to the elbow. Repeat rhythmically for several minutes. Then do step four on the right arm.

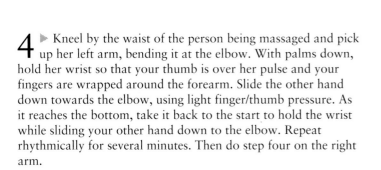

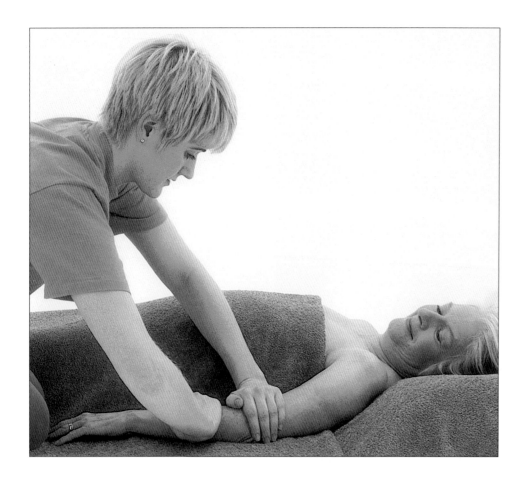

5 ◄ With her arm down by her side, place your hands, palms down, around her left wrist with your fingers pointing in opposite directions. Push both hands up the arm, slowly and deeply, to the shoulder. Curve your top hand over and back under the shoulder, then slide both hands lightly down the sides of the arm from shoulder to fingers. Repeat rhythmically for several minutes, then start again, this time working on the right arm.

6 ► The person being massaged should turn over so that she is lying face down and you should kneel by her toes. Do a full leg stroke. Start with palms down, one hand on the sole of each foot, fingers pointing inwards. Then with a slow, firm pressure, push up the sole of the foot, over the heel, up the calf, gently over the knee, then up the thigh and sides of buttocks to finish at the hips. Repeat ten times, moving up the body as you push slowly and firmly.

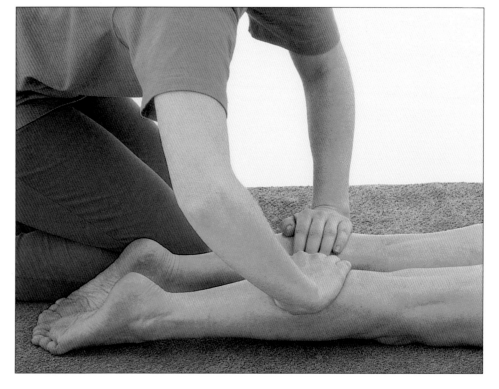

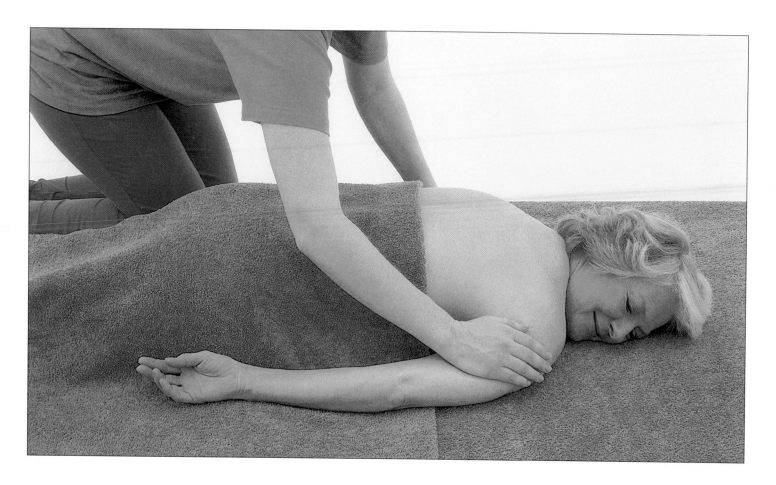

7 ▲ Kneeling by her waist, place her hands at her sides. Do a full arm stroke. Start with your palms over hers, fingers pointing upwards. Using a medium pressure, slowly push your hands up her arms, gently over the elbow, and across the shoulders to finish at the neck. Repeat ten times, bending so you move up the body as you push slowly and firmly, keeping the pressure even throughout.

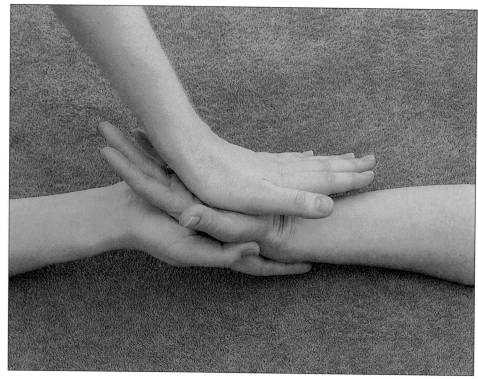

8 ▶ Pick up one hand, palm upwards, and sandwich it between yours. Do a short, fast, firm friction rub from fingertips to wrist for several minutes. Finish off by pressing your hands in to squeeze hers for a count of ten, then slowly slide your fingers down and off the tips of hers. Repeat all of step eight on the other hand.

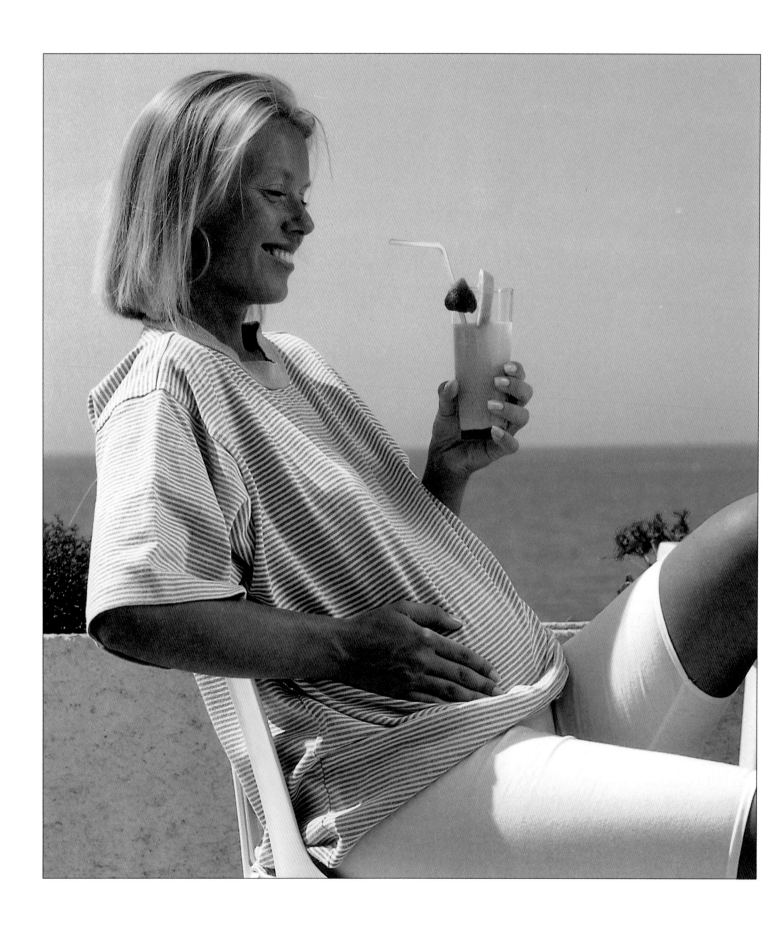

THE ANTI-STRETCH MARK MASSAGE

✳

When you put on weight – either during pregnancy or from over-eating – the skin has to stretch enormously to encompass the enlarged you. This often causes stretch marks, the fine white lines like snails' trails across the skin, which are, in fact, tiny scars in the underlying tissue. They occur most often on the thighs, stomach and bottom, but can sometimes appear on breasts or upper arms.

Unfortunately, once you have them, they are almost impossible to get rid of. However, if you gently massage in a rich oil, such as wheatgerm, jojoba or sweet almond, you can gradually improve the texture and tone of skin, help the white marks fade quicker and reduce the likelihood of over-stretching occurring again.

The anti-stretch mark massage is ideal to use as a preventative measure. If you do it every day, it will help skin stretch as far as it needs to and then return to normal. So steps one to four are specifically designed to be used throughout pregnancy right up to term. Steps five to eight are to be done as a post-natal massage. However, the entire routine may be used when you are not pregnant and is also ideal for anyone who knows she should be dieting but has not quite got round to doing it yet.

HOW TO DO AN ANTI-STRETCH MARK MASSAGE

If you are pregnant, the best position is lying on your back propped up on pillows so that you are half sitting. However, if you are near term, you will probably find it uncomfortable to lie on your back for any length of time, so instead turn on your side and lie with your knees bent. For anyone else, lie stretched out, face up.

The movements in this massage are slow, soothing, with lots of repetitions to push oil into skin. Use plenty of oil and once it is absorbed, add more – this is the one massage where you can end up looking like a sardine! Do not press down into the abdomen during any strokes and keep all movements on the tummy light and as gentle as possible.

(Left) Prevent stretch marks during and after pregnancy with gentle massage techniques.

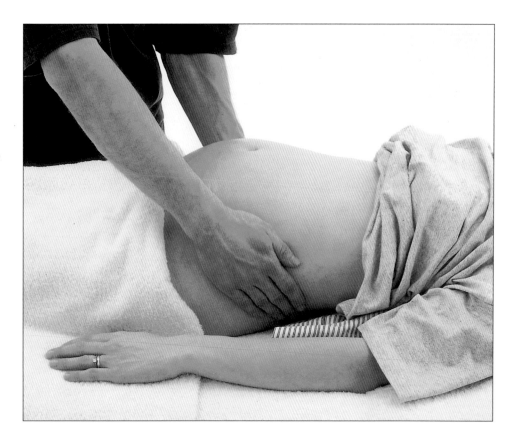

WARNING
During pregnancy be gentle with all massage strokes and *never* push/press down into the abdomen.

This anti-stretch mark massage is ideal to use as a preventative measure. Steps 1–4 are designed to be used throughout pregnancy right up to term. Steps 5–8 are to be done as a post-natal massage.

1 ◀ Place your hands, palms down, at the base of the ribs over the solar plexus, with your fingers pointing up to the chest. Draw your hands out to the sides, then pull them down the waist more firmly and gently round over the hips to stop below the navel. Repeat for several minutes, using the stroke as a gentle way to warm and spread the oil.

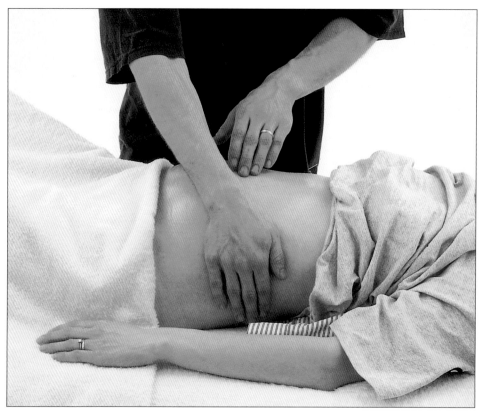

2 ▶ Do a firm side stroke up the waist. With hands, palms down against the top of one thigh, tuck your fingers as far as possible down under the bottom. Pull hands up the sides of the torso, one after the other, in a smooth, flowing stroke. Work from the thigh up to the base of the ribs for several minutes. Then repeat on the other side of the body.

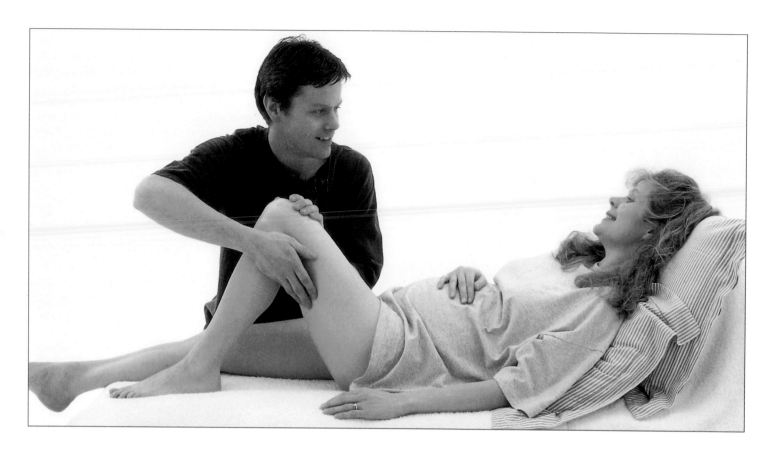

3 ▲ Bend one leg up at the knee and then do some firm, sweeping strokes up the leg. Place the palms of your hands above the knee and push up to the thigh, with one hand following the other. Keep going for several minutes. Then do the same stroke on the inner and outer sides of the thigh, taking the outer stroke up to the hip. Repeat on the other leg.

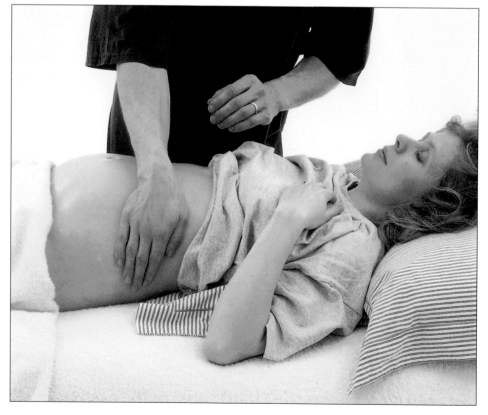

4 ▶ Lightly place your right hand, palm down, at the base of the ribs over the solar plexus. Make large, gentle, sweeping circles in a clockwise direction right around the abdomen for several minutes. Then repeat the stroke, this time using both hands so that one follows the other in a smooth, flowing motion, clockwise around the tummy.

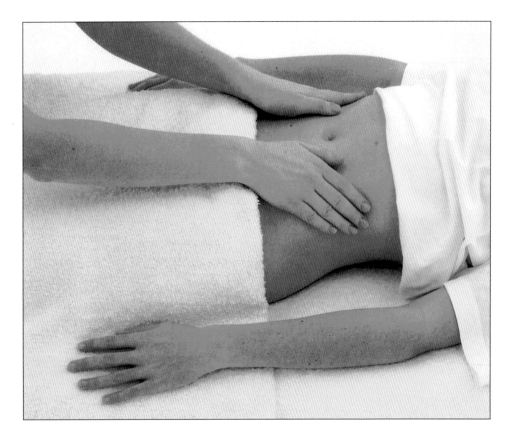

5 ◄ Place both hands, palms down, below the navel, with your thumbs together and palms slightly raised so that only the fingers make contact with the tummy. Gently slide your hands upwards and let your fingers glide out to the sides below the ribs and down the sides of the waist pulling firmly, then lightly round and back to the start. Continue the stroke for several minutes.

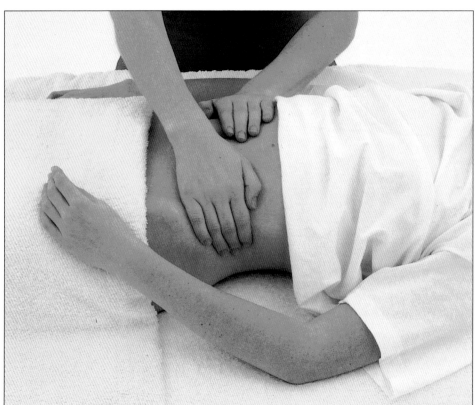

6 ▶ Place one hand, palm down, on either side of the waist. Then firmly pull both hands up the sides in unison, moving them across the tummy to the opposite side of the waist. Repeat continuously, so that your hands criss-cross back and forth over the abdomen.

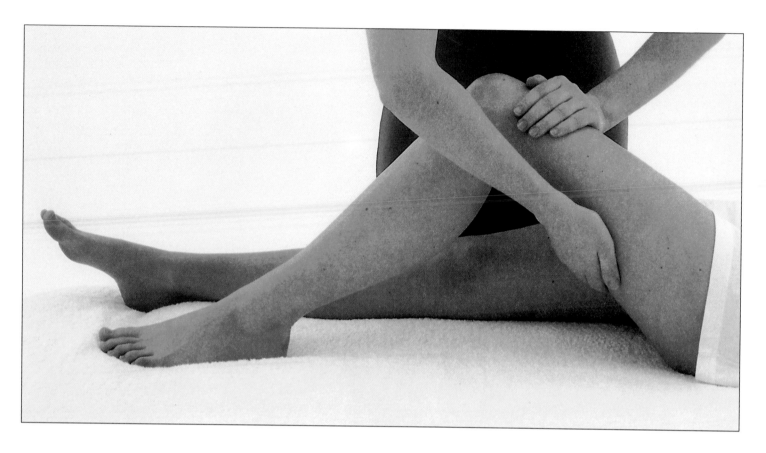

7 ▲ Bend the leg at the knee again. Wrap your right hand, palm up, around the back of the thigh, thumb to the outer and fingers to the inner sides. Start with your hand just behind the knee, then firmly push in and squeeze slightly as you slide your hand up the thigh muscle to the buttock. Repeat the movement continuously, using only the right hand, for several minutes.

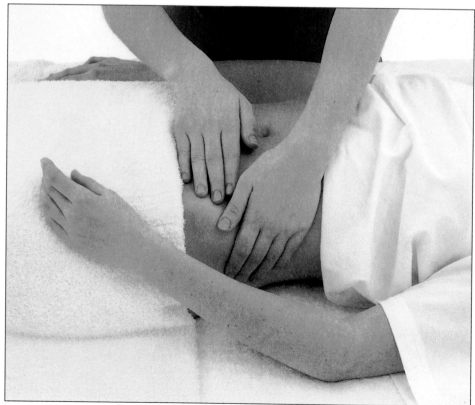

8 ▶ Place both hands, palms down, on the tummy, one between the base of the ribs and the other below the navel. Make a large circle around the abdomen in a clockwise direction, with one hand doing one half of the circle and the other completing it, as a smooth, flowing stroke. Repeat, with one hand on top of the other, and make full circles that get slower and slower.

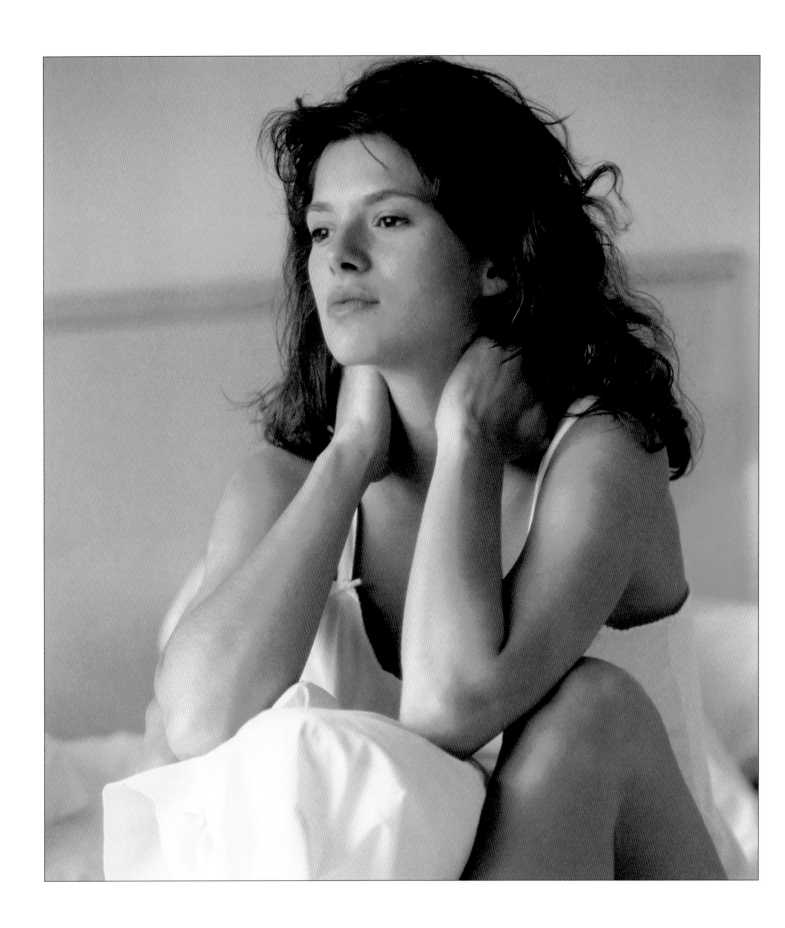

MASSAGE TO SOOTHE PMT & PERIOD PAIN

Premenstrual Tension and period pain are not really ailments that can be cured. They are just things women have learned to live with, particularly as the symptoms recur every month, regular as clockwork. If you are unlucky enough to suffer from either complaint, then you know how easily they can turn you from a pussycat into a tiger.

They affect your mind, so you can burst into tears, be irrational, irritable, depressed, lethargic or crave sweet foods all in the same day. They make your body bloated and spotty, with back ache or cramps that feel as if you are wearing an iron girdle.

Unfortunately, massage does not wipe away all of these symptoms. It can certainly make you feel better, feel pampered and feel more like a pussycat again. It can also reduce the bloated feeling of your swollen abdomen and soothe cramps and the nagging lower back ache that seems to drag you down all day.

As everything from the waist down seems to feel tender during a bad period, the strokes in this massage are all gentle, light and soothing. If you feel you need a firmer touch, particularly for the lower back pain, try the massage specifically for that on page 88. Or if it is a month when you have little discomfort but feel very, very bloated, try the anti-cellulite massage on page 61 instead.

HOW TO SOOTHE PMT AND PERIOD PAIN

It is important to soothe the mind as much as the body, so this is a good massage to have while playing your favourite music and lying in a dimly lit room with the door locked to keep away the world (which includes children or pets!). If it makes you feel better, have a box of chocolates close to hand.

Use plenty of oil so your hands slip easily as this is not meant to be a deep or firm massage. The lighter the strokes, the more soothing they feel and do as many repeats as possible.

(Left) Lethargy and depression strike some women every month.

1 ▶ Steps one to five are done with the person being massaged lying face down. Place your hands, palms down, on either side of the spine near the tailbone, 5 cm (2 inches) away from it. Push your hands up and fan them smoothly out to the sides at the waist, then pull them down the torso and across the buttocks to the start position. Repeat for several minutes, using this stroke to pull and push flesh up, round and down.

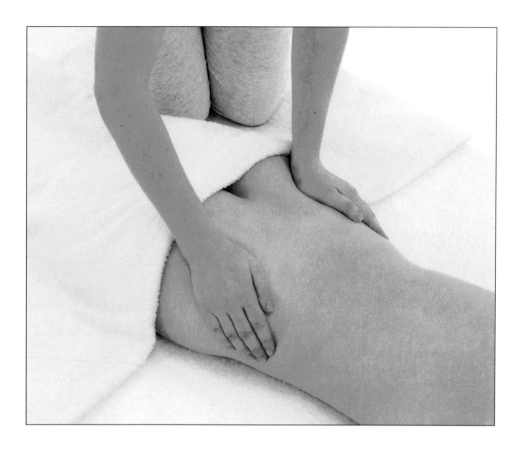

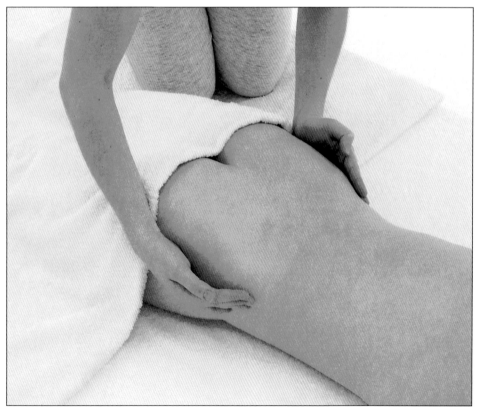

2 ◀ Place hands, palms down, on either side of the top of the waist. Using the heels of your hands and the little fingers, press firmly in as you slide your hands down to the hips, then draw them into either side of the spine. Slide your hands up the middle of the back, still using the heels and little fingers for the stroke, then fan them out to the top of the waist. Repeat for several minutes.

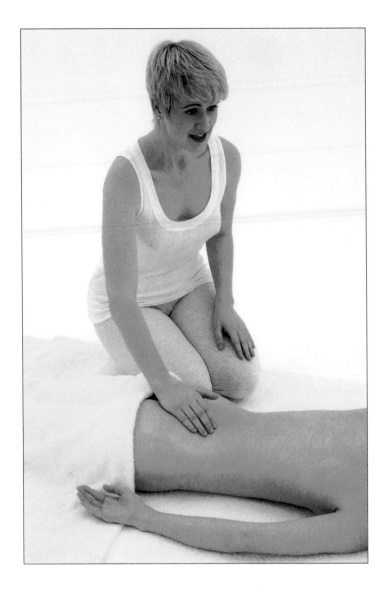

3 ◄ Place the palm of your right hand over the tailbone (sacrum) and use pressure from the heel of the hand to stroke around in circles. Then place the heels of your hands on either side of the tailbone and slowly push up the length of the spine to the waist, then lightly glide your hands back down. Repeat the entire stroke for several minutes.

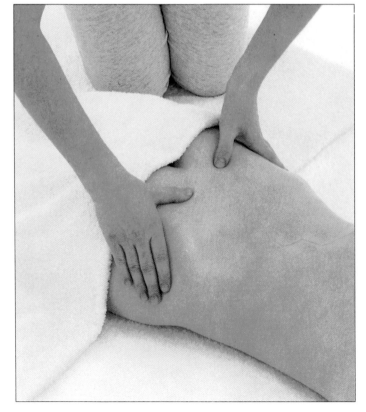

4 ▶ Using your thumbs only, make small circles to knead all the way up the lower back. Start with them 5 cm (2 inches) out from either side of the tailbone and slowly work up the spine to the waist. Repeat several times. Then place your hands, palms down, under each hip and pull the flesh up with your fingers into the middle of the lower back. Repeat as a smooth, flowing stroke.

5 ▶ Knead one side of the torso, from the top of the thigh up to the waist. Use the thumb and fingers of both hands to pinch, twist and squeeze the flesh, with your hands working in unison. Repeat on the other side of the torso. Then, repeat the same kneading stroke across the top of the buttocks and up the middle of the lower back to the waistline.

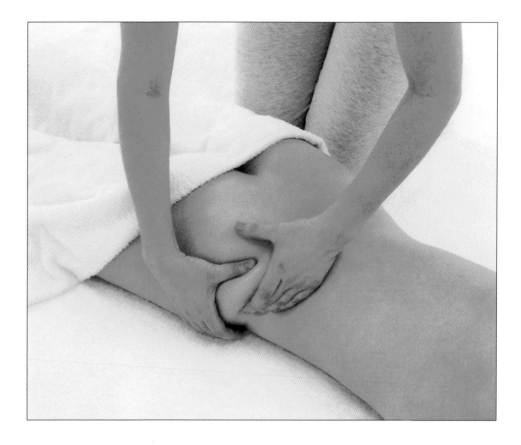

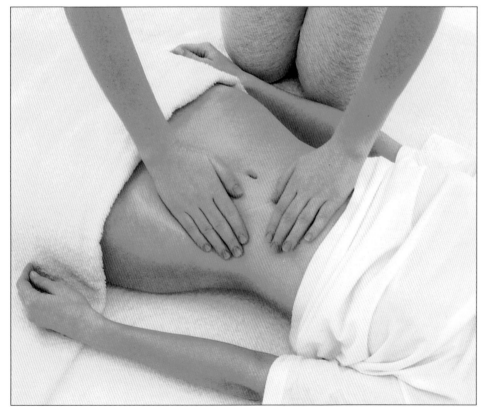

6 ◀ The person being massaged should turn so that she is lying face up. Place your left hand over her solar plexus at the base of the ribs, and leave it there throughout the stroke. Place your right hand, palm down, above the navel and make large clockwise circles down one side, across the groin and up to the start position. Keep the stroke light, gentle and rhythmic for several minutes.

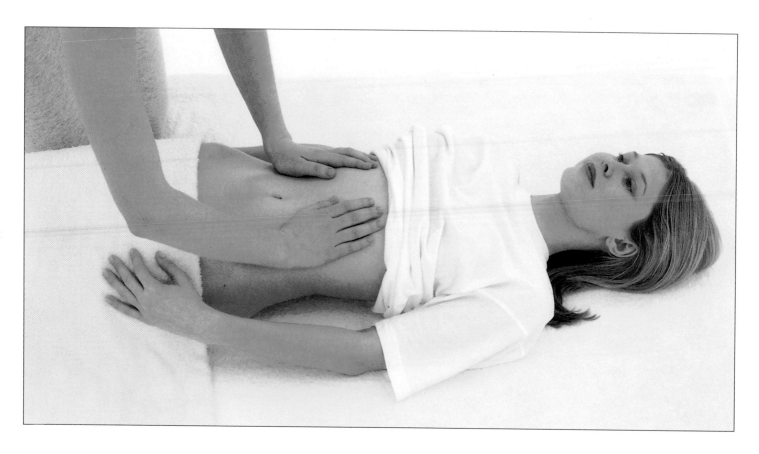

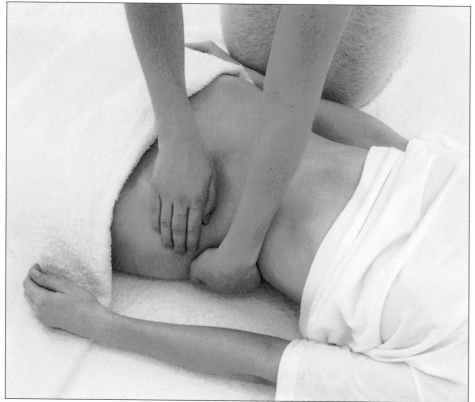

7 ▲ Place both hands, palms down, over the solar plexus at the base of the ribs, with your fingers pointing upwards. Slowly fan your hands out to the sides, slide them firmly down the waist, sweep them round under the navel them gently slide them up the tummy to the start. Repeat for several minutes, keeping the stroke smooth and flowing throughout.

8 ◄ Place your hands, palms down, on one side of the waist, with your fingers tucked well under the back. With one hand following the other, firmly pull the flesh up towards the navel, working from the top of the thigh to the top of the waist. Then gently bend the knees of the person being massaged up to her chest, with your hands pressing down at the top of her shins. Hold for a count of ten, relax and repeat.

59

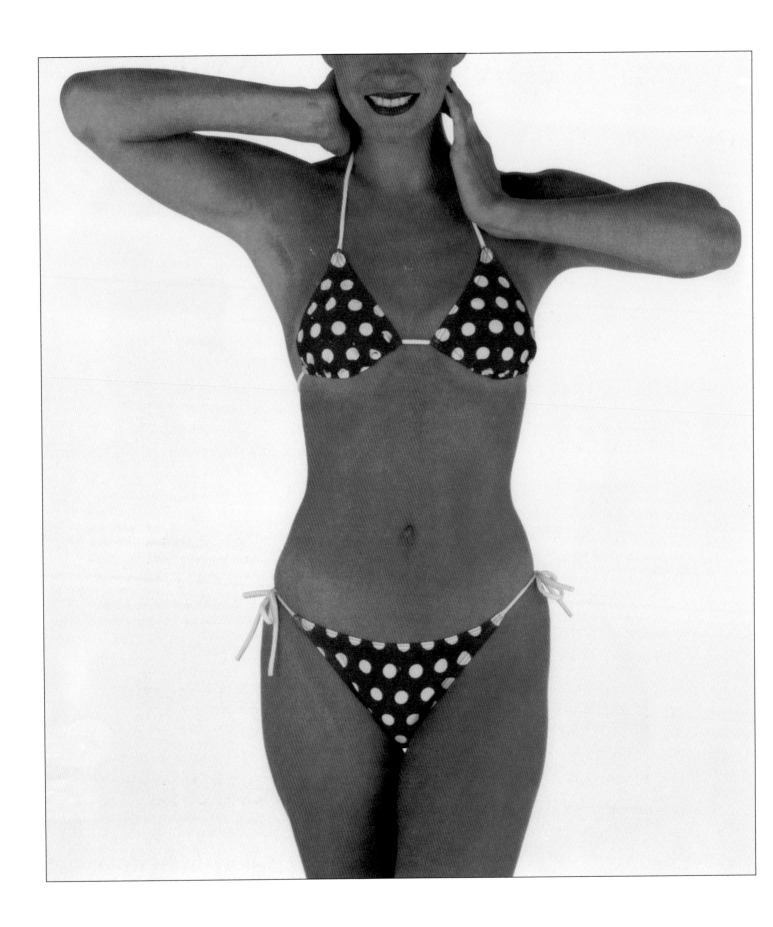

ANTI-CELLULITE MASSAGE

Ask almost any doctor about cellulite and he will say that there is no such thing, but ask 90 per cent of women and they will show you living proof of its existence – mainly on their upper legs, buttocks or tummy.

Cellulite is a word that the beauty industry uses to explain the dimpled, lumpy areas of fat that appear just below the skin. Until recently, the experts thought it was exclusive to women and that female hormones caused the unusual fat deposits. However, the latest research from cosmetic companies proves that men have cellulite too, only it is not so near the surface and so does not show as lumps under the skin.

This has led to a new theory on exactly what causes cellulite. It seems likely that toxic wastes, that are not flushed out of the body due to poor circulation and lack of exercise, cause a chemical reaction which puts a hard coating around the normally soft fat cells. This is why they become lumpy and the skin dimples. It is also why cellulite appears in areas where circulation is slow – such as the bottom, which we sit on too much!

While the cosmetic industry looks for new ingredients to stop this chemical reaction, anything that speeds up the circulation in areas of cellulite or helps break up the hard rim of these fat cells will improve areas of cellulite. Massage can do both – the friction brings fresh blood to the skin surface, while the warmth and rubbing action help break down the rims around the fat cells. So this massage is specifically designed to include lots of vigorous movements which leave skin tingling and rosy with oxygenated blood.

HOW TO DO AN ANTI-CELLULITE MASSAGE

This is a do-it-yourself massage, since few of us willingly expose our cellulite once we have a good store of it! Steps one to four are best done sitting with your knees bent. Steps five to eight should be done standing, although you can put your foot up on a chair or on the side of a bath if it makes it easier.

For best results, do the massage morning and night using lots of oil or a favourite cream. Always do all strokes in an upwards direction, towards the heart, to help get the blood flowing and stop body toxins building up.

(Left) Regular anti-cellulite massage will improve the appearance of cellulite within weeks.

1 ▶ For steps one to four, sit comfortably bending the knee of the leg you are working on. Start with the right leg and stroke firmly up the thigh from knee to hip, with one hand following the other in a flowing motion. Do the entire thigh – inner, outer, front and back.

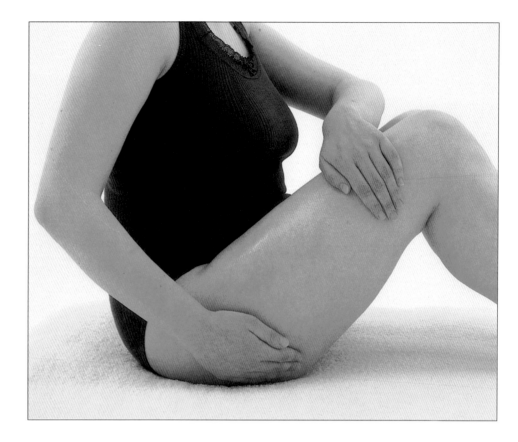

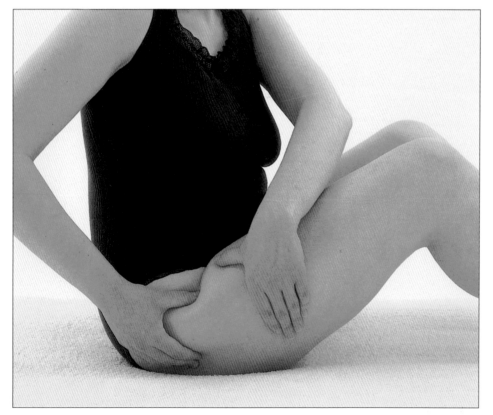

2 ◀ Knead the thigh all over, pinching and squeezing flesh between the thumbs and fingers of both hands. Again, start from above the knee and work in an upwards direction to the top of the thigh. The hands should work together, with one pointing down and the other upwards.

3 ▶ Bend your fingers stiffly at the first joint and firmly drag your hands from the knee up the thigh, rolling them under so the knuckles also rake the skin as you pull your hands upwards. One hand should follow after the other. Be gentle on the outer thigh as knuckling can hurt.

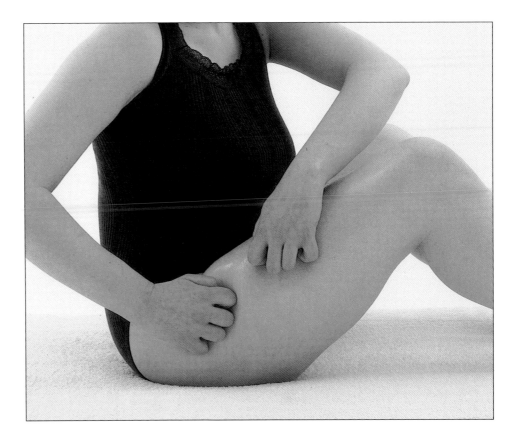

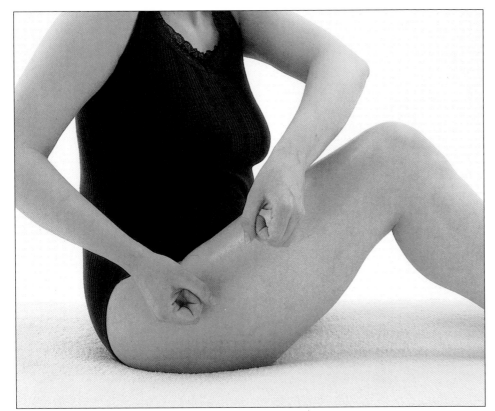

4 ◀ Make your hands into loose, relaxed fists and use them to pummel all over the thigh by tapping down and bouncing up quickly and lightly. Use the flat part of your fists from the first joint to the fingertips, so your hands are hitting palm down, one after the other.

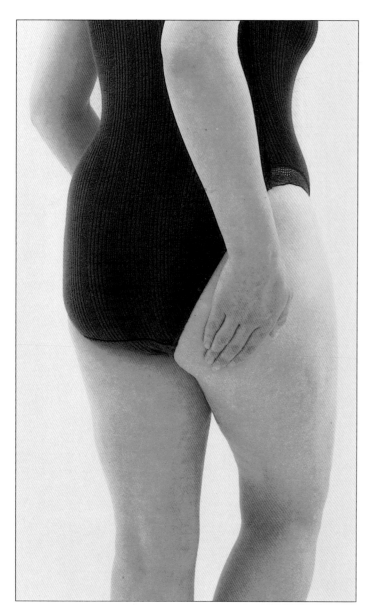

5 ◀ Stand up while doing steps five to eight. Place your right hand, palm down, on your right buttock and make large, firm, flowing circles keeping your hand flat. Start on the hip and move clockwise down to the thigh and back round the cheek of the buttock to the start.

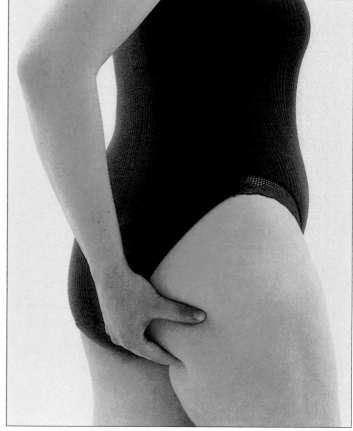

6 ▶ Standing and using the same hand, knead the right buttock muscle, using your thumb and fingers in a pinching, squeezing movement. Begin where the thigh meets the curve of the buttock and work upwards to the hip, wherever there is loose flesh. Try to make firm, fast movements.

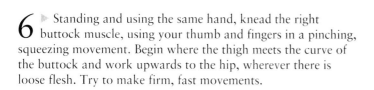

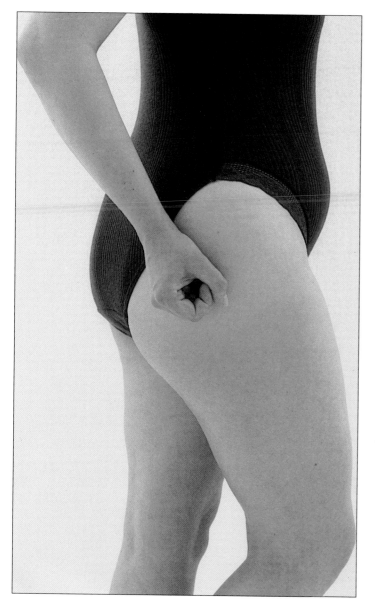

7 ◄ Make your right hand into a loose, relaxed fist and use it to pummel all over the right buttock by tapping down and bouncing up quickly and lightly. Use the flat part of your fist from the first joint to the fingertips, so that your hand is hitting palm down, and work in an upwards direction.

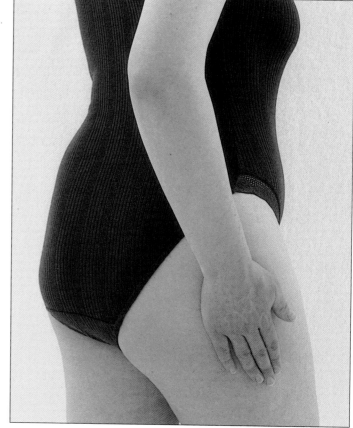

8 ▶ Finish off with long, smooth, deep strokes, using one hand after the other, from mid-thigh up over the buttock to the hip. Use the flat of your hand, in a friction rub, moving the hand up and down in short, fast sawing movements. Now repeat all steps on the left side.

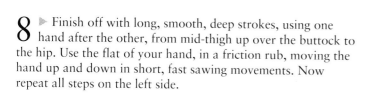

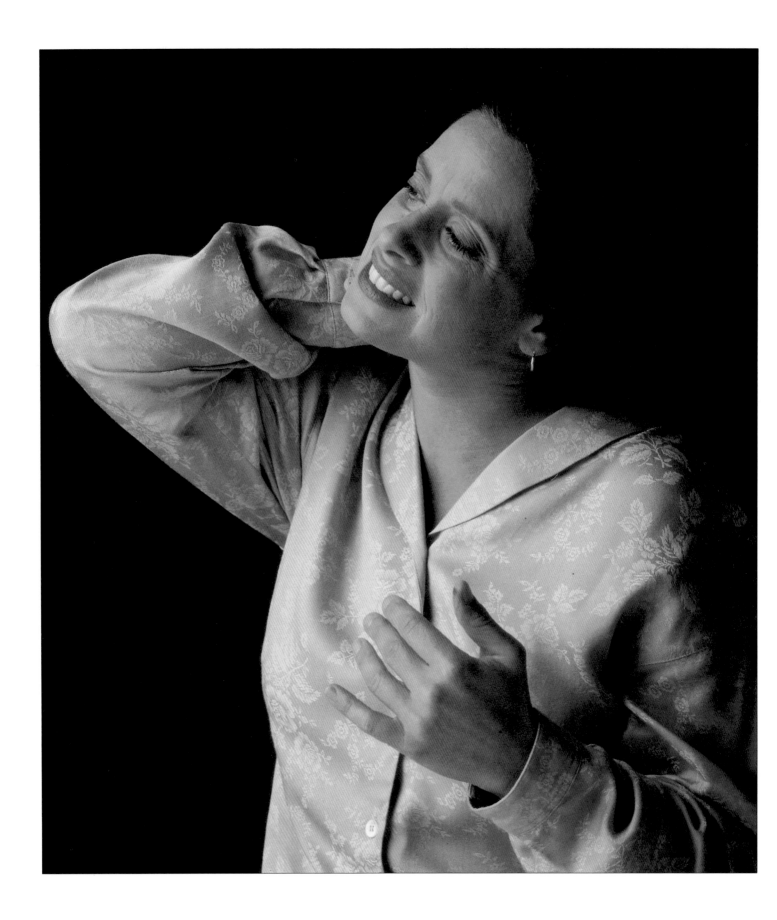

MASSAGE TO RELIEVE A STIFF NECK

A stiff neck can be caused by anything from stress or sitting in a draught, to sleeping in an odd position or watching too many games of tennis. It is, literally, a complete pain in the neck and it makes the simplest task, such as reversing into a car parking space, a slow and excruciating torture. It also makes you realize how many times you move your head in a normal day. If you have children, you soon discover how much easier it is to nod a 'Yes' than it is to shake a 'No'!

A stiff neck is also one of the simplest ailments to cure and two things help tremendously – heat and massage. So the best kind of neck massage uses lots of simple movements with plenty of warming repetitions, plus some deep kneading strokes to relax and release any areas with trapped nerves or muscle tension.

This one not only does that, but it is also so simple that you can do it anywhere. As it is done with the sufferer sitting upright, you can even massage someone at work, while she leans forward onto her desk, fully clothed.

It brings instant relief, but stiff neck muscles do have a nasty habit of coming back during the night, so it is best to have a long soak in a warm, deep bath as soon after the massage (and before bed) as possible. Alternatively, at the end of the massage, rub a product containing menthol up the sides of the neck so that it warms the skin and muscles for some time afterwards.

HOW TO MASSAGE A STIFF NECK

The best position for this massage is for the sufferer to be seated on a comfortable, upright chair. For steps one to four, she should lean forward onto a cushion resting on a table, or sit facing the back of the chair and prop the cushion between her and the chair back.

If possible, she should wear a towel and you should use lots of oil so that your hands really slip over the sore neck muscles. If the sufferer needs to be fully clothed, keep your movements light over any tender areas.

(Left) Heat and massage are simple ways to bring instant relief to an aching neck.

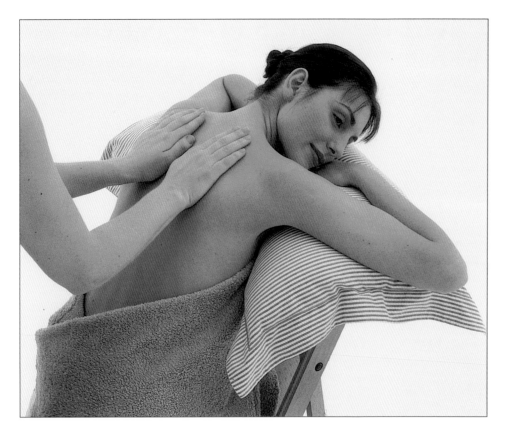

1 ◀ Place your hands, palms down, on either side of the spine in the middle of the back. With a firm pressure, push you hands up to the shoulder tops, then slide one hand out on each side to the top of the arm, draw them back in across the top of the shoulders and up either side of the neck. Repeat the stroke from start to finish for several minutes, using it to feel for any tense spots of knotted muscles as you go.

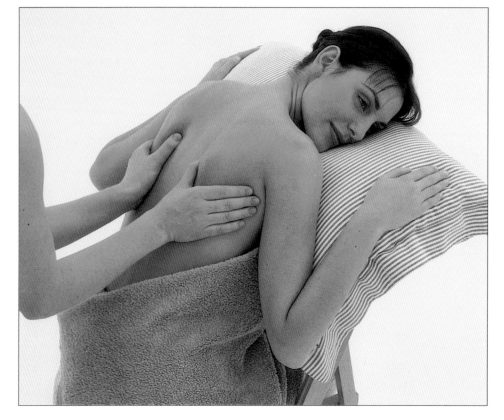

2 ▶ Start with the sufferer bending forward onto the pillow, so that her shoulder blades protrude. With flat, straight hands, place the sides of the palms and the little fingers across the top of the shoulder muscle and do a firm, fast friction rub across the muscle from arm to neck. Repeat on the other side. Then using your thumbs only, make small circles to knead under the shoulder blades and up the spine to the top of the neck.

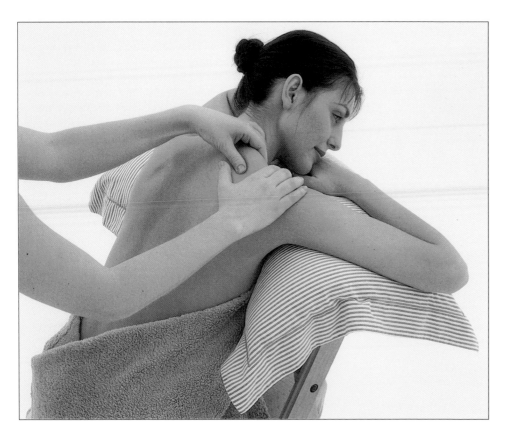

3 ◄ With your fingers forward, place your hands, palms down, over each shoulder muscle by the sides of the neck. Push and pull the shoulder top muscle back and forth. Then working on one side with both hands, squeeze, pinch and knead the muscle for several minutes. Finish by standing on the opposite side, placing palms over the top of the arm and sweep the hands up the side of the neck, one after the other.

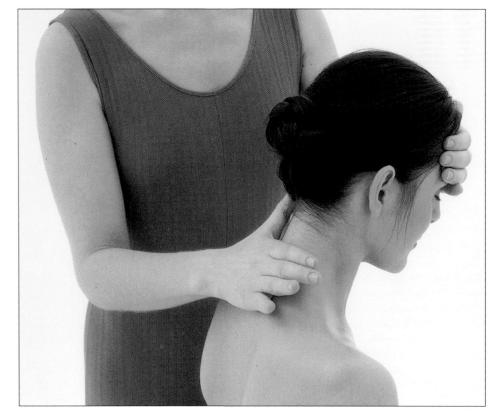

4 ► Hold the base of the sufferer's neck with your thumb to the right and fingers to the left and support her head as she bends forward. Rub your hand quickly up and down the neck in a very light friction stroke for two minutes. Then roll your hand across the neck from left to right and back, to push and pull the muscles against the vertebrae. Make sure you have plenty of oil for both strokes and keep the pressure light over areas of muscle stiffness.

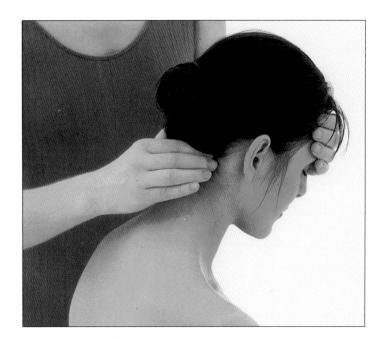

5 ◄ Place the palm of your left hand on the sufferer's
forehead and use it to support her head as she bends
forward. Place the thumb of your right hand on one side of the
last vertebrae at the top of the neck, and the index finger on the
other side. Press in with the tips of thumb and finger and hold
for a count of ten, then release and make small circles over the
same area. Repeat, working in a line outwards, across the skull
from ear to ear.

6 ▶ Make the sufferer sit upright, with
shoulders straight but relaxed. Place
your hands, palms down, around her arm
tops with your fingers forward. Gently
push her shoulders forwards until you
feel a stretch and hold for a count of ten.
Relax. Then, with your hands in the same
position, gently pull her shoulders back
and hold the stretch for a count of ten.
Repeat both stretches, forwards and
backwards.

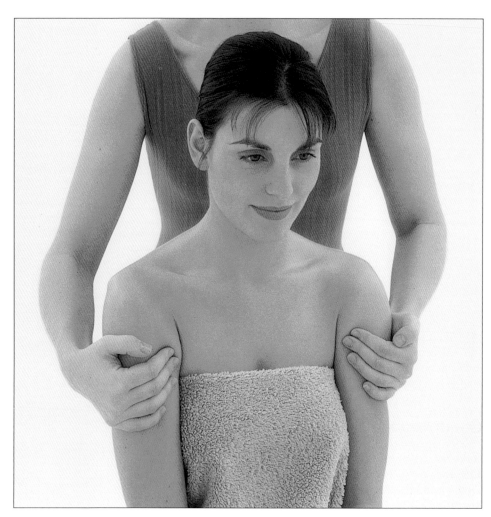

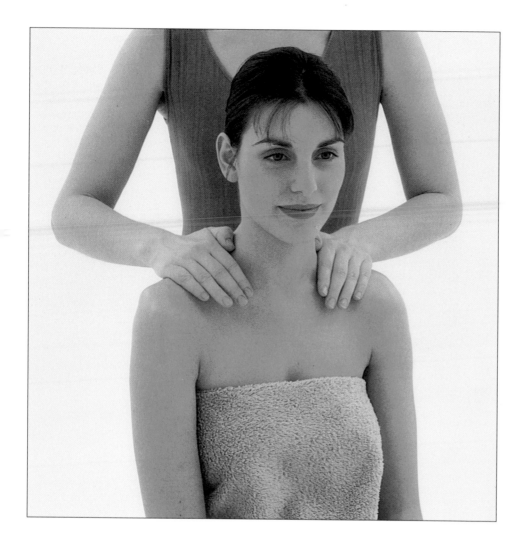

7 ◄ In the same position, place the palms of your hands down on the shoulders, on either side of the neck, with fingers pointing forwards. Push down firmly with your hands while the sufferer slowly drops her head back as far as is comfortable. Hold for a count of ten, then get her to raise her head to the upright position and release the downward pressure of your hands. Repeat twice more from the beginning.

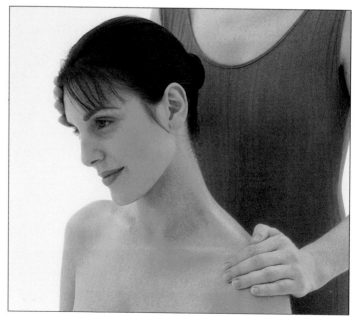

8 ▶ While she is sitting upright, bend her head to the right side and support it with your right hand, palm up above her ear. Place your left hand below her other ear, with your thumb under the jaw and fingers stretched round the nape of the neck. Slide your hand down the length of the neck and across the shoulder top to the arm, pressing down to stretch the muscle. Repeat several times on both sides of the neck.

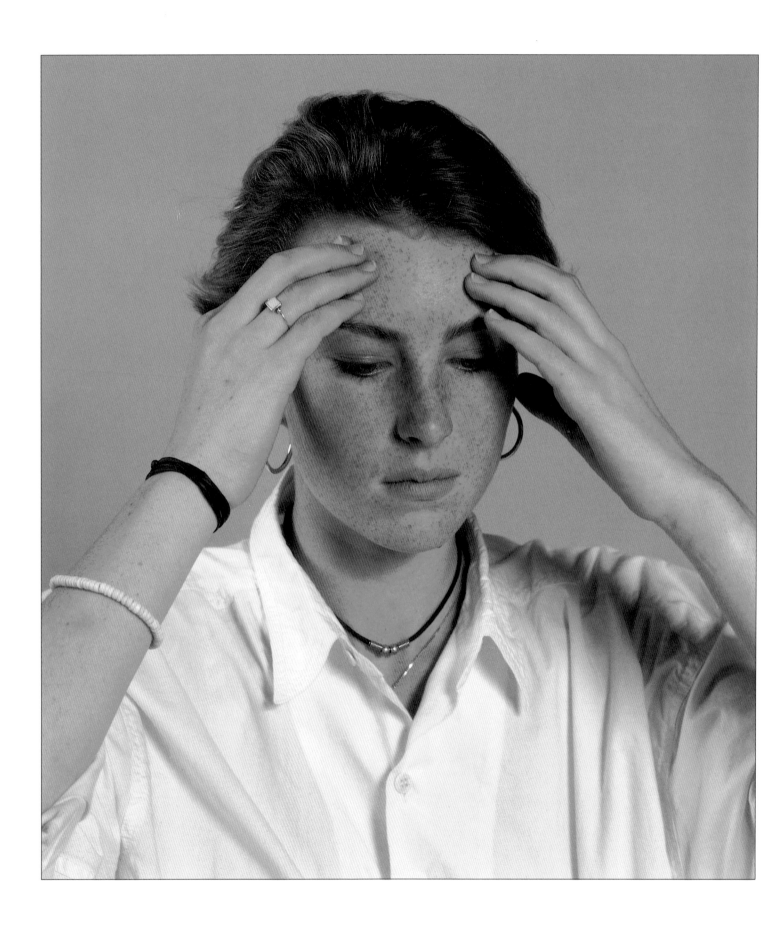

TENSION HEADACHE MASSAGE

❋

Every thought you think, every worry, every anxiety, every problem, scowl, glower or frown ends up on the poor old head. The web of tiny muscles from the neck take up the strain, knotting and tightening into a full-blown headache.

The best way to take this weight off your shoulders is with a soothing face, neck and scalp massage. Not only does it instantly relieve the tight, tense, aching muscles, but it also relaxes the over-tired, overwrought mind. As you massage away the headache and its source, you also release a lot of stress from the rest of the body and will feel calm, tranquil and deeply relaxed all over. In fact, this simple massage has been known to make even a total workaholic stretch out immediately afterwards for a quiet snooze.

To be effective you need the time for lots of slow, soothing repetitions of all the strokes. The more you do it, the better it feels. However, you can find out exactly where the headache seems worse – temples, scalp, eyes, forehead or neck – and spend extra time in this area.

If you have persistent, recurrent headaches always seek medical advice, as they may be caused by something other than stress.

HOW TO MASSAGE AN ACHING HEAD

The best position is lying on your back, as comfortably as possible, with your head supported on a flat pillow or folded towel. To keep any strain off your lower back and to help you relax while lying face up, place another pillow under your knees so that they are bent. Also, have extra towels or blankets ready for warmth, and wear something that leaves the shoulders bare.

A dimly lit or darkened room is very soothing, particularly if you have been in bright light (welding, sunshine, etc.) or flickering light (fluorescent tubes, computer screens, etc.) for several hours beforehand. To keep everything as quiet as possible, take the telephone off the hook, throw pets and children outside, close the door firmly and reach for the oil!

(Left) By the end of a busy day it may feel as if you are wearing a hat made from cement.

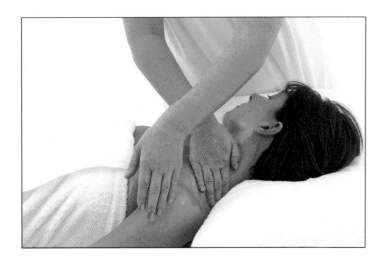

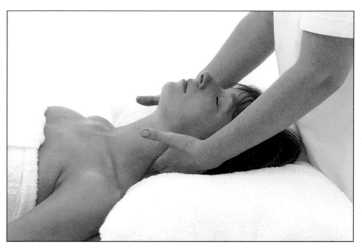

1 ▲ Oil your hands well. Place both palms over the upper arm near one shoulder and slowly pull one hand up the neck towards the ears, followed by the other hand, gently stretching the neck muscles. Repeat several times in a smooth, firm stroking movement. Repeat on the other side. Then slide your hands under the top of the back, low between the shoulder blades and, using a very firm stroke, pull up, sliding one hand after the other up to the nape of the neck. Repeat several times.

2 ▲ Place your hands under the nape of the neck (between the shoulders and skull) and gently stretch the neck upwards 3-5 cm (1-2 inches) to arch it until you feel resistance. Do not lift the head off the cushion. Hold for a count of five, then gently and slowly release the neck. Repeat, stretching and lowering the neck at the same speed three times without any jerky movements. It is important to support the neck across flat fingertips, so that you do not press inwards.

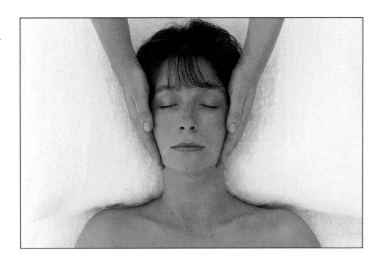

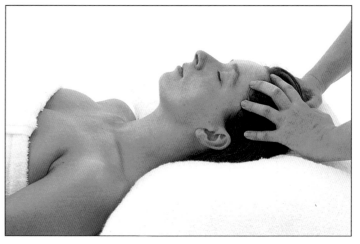

3 ▲ With your fingers and hand cupping the chin, gently pull up the sides of the cheeks, pressing in over the temples until your hands meet above the eyebrows. Pull your palms back, one after the other, in a firm stroke up to the top of the head. Finish by pressing the top and sides of the head between your hands and hold for a count of five. Repeat several times, trying to let all the movements flow in a gentle, soothing, full-face stroke from beginning to end.

4 ▲ Keeping your fingers stiff, place the pads of your fingertips on the scalp all around the hairline. Using the lightest inwards pressure, make tiny circles with your fingers in the same position so that you rotate the scalp for a count of ten. The movement is similar to shampooing your hair – but a rubbing, rolling motion rather than scrubbing. Repeat, repositioning your fingers farther back until you end up at the crown. Then repeat round the hairline at the nape of the neck.

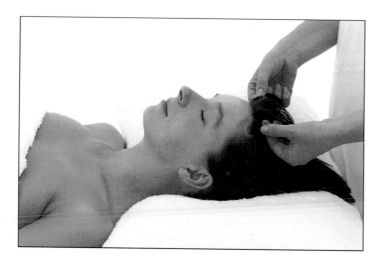

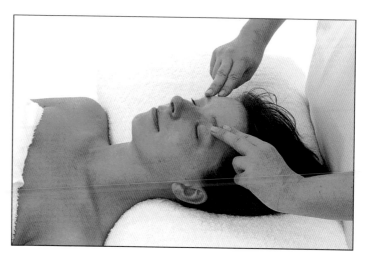

5 ▲ Now run your fingers through the hair, drawing it away from the head in a soothing stroke, for a minute or more. Take a small section of hair between finger and thumb, and tug it repeatedly and firmly for a count of five. If you hold the hair section as close to the roots as possible this will not hurt. Repeat all over the head – this gives an instant boost to the blood circulation and relaxes the scalp in one go. Finish by pushing in with your hands and squeezing the head all over.

6 ▲ Place your fingertips gently over the eyelids and, using the tiniest amount of downward pressure, hold for a count of five, then relax for a count of five. Repeat twice. Stroke from the middle to the outer eyebrows firmly, using the tips of your first two fingers, in a slow, steady movement. Repeat several times. Using the same fingers, make slow circles over the temples so that the skin rotates, then slide them up into the hairline.

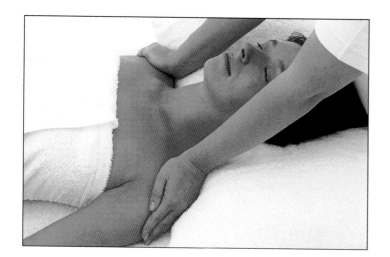

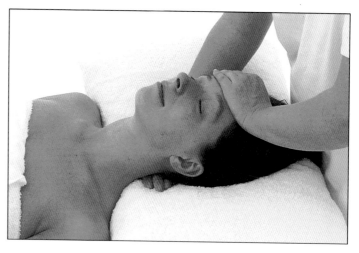

7 ▲ To release shoulder and neck tension, place one palm over the top of the rounded part of each shoulder. Gently press down to open up the chest, holding the shoulders back for a count of five. Relax and repeat again. Then slide your hands under and push the shoulders upwards and round them into the chest to release the upper back and neck support muscles. Hold for a count of five, relax, then repeat.

8 ▲ Finish off with a deeply relaxing, slow stroke. Place your left hand palm down on the forehead and your right hand palm up under the back of the neck. Push inwards gently with both hands as you draw them slowly up the head until they meet at the crown. The lower hand must gently lift and tilt the head as part of the stroke. Repeat this stroke as many times as you like, getting slower and gentler each time.

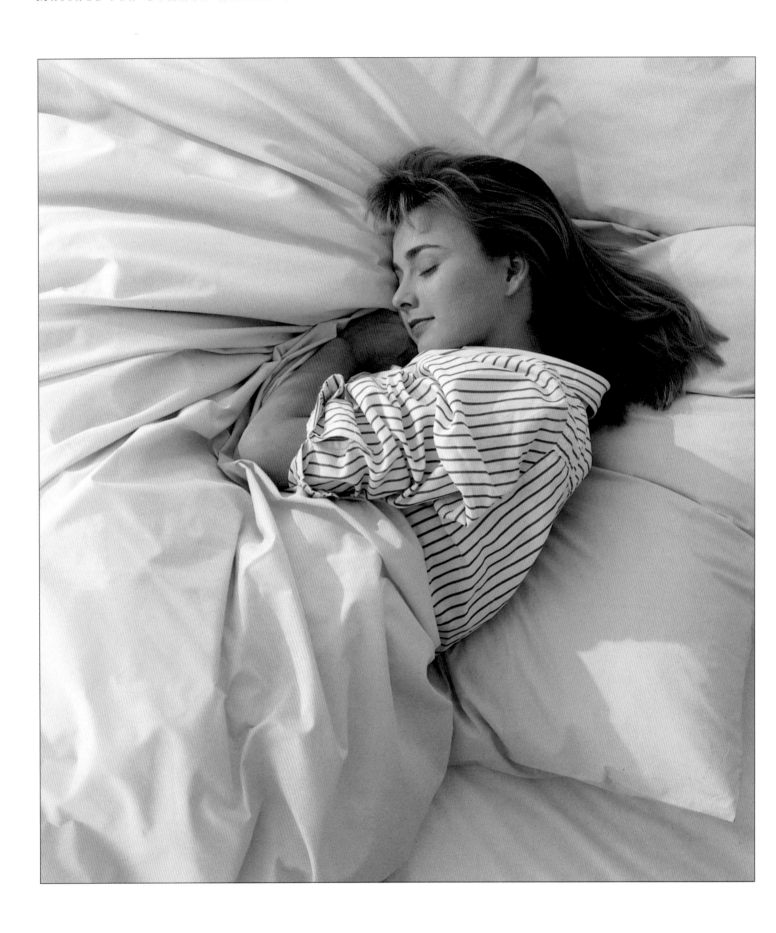

MASSAGE FOR SLEEPLESSNESS

Anyone who has ever had a sleepless night knows that counting sheep is no help at all. Neither is a hot, milky drink, late-night television or a bad book. Sometimes, even a sleeping tablet does not work.

As you pace the floor, hour after hour, baggy-eyed but wide awake, the tension mounts because insomnia is one of the most irritating, frustrating and stressful ailments known. If your muscles were hanging loose before bedtime, after several hours of tossing and turning they will be tense, taut and totally uptight. The more frustrated you are at not being able to sleep, the less likely you are to sleep anyway.

A long soak in a very warm bath, followed by a slow, soothing massage is the one thing that usually has a Rip van Winkle effect – and even if it does not put you to sleep, it makes you feel a lot better about being awake! Most insomniacs are over-stimulated, so it is important to use massage strokes that sweep over large areas of the body to loosen knotted muscles. This, combined with simple stretches to release trapped tension, invariably has the desired effect, and if muscles are relaxed, sleep is possible.

This massage for sleeplessness uses friction rubs and muscle flexes for fast, total relaxation. It is best to do it after a warm bath and before your usual bedtime so that you are relaxed and ready for sleep. However, if you must do it in the wee hours of the night – and you know someone kind enough to stay awake and massage you – at least it is speedy and simple to do.

HOW TO MASSAGE THE SLEEPLESS

You need lots of pillows, soft lighting, layers of snug blankets, warm hands and plenty of warm oil. Comfort is vital so that the poor insomniac relaxes and, as you want him to go to sleep, bed is the best place to do the massage.

Keep all movements light and rhythmic to warm and relax the body as quickly as possible. The more repetitions of strokes the better, so each one can get slower and gentler towards the end. Do steps one to five with the person being massaged lying face down, and steps six to eight with him face up.

(Left) Tense muscles are certain to keep sleep at bay, so massage is the answer.

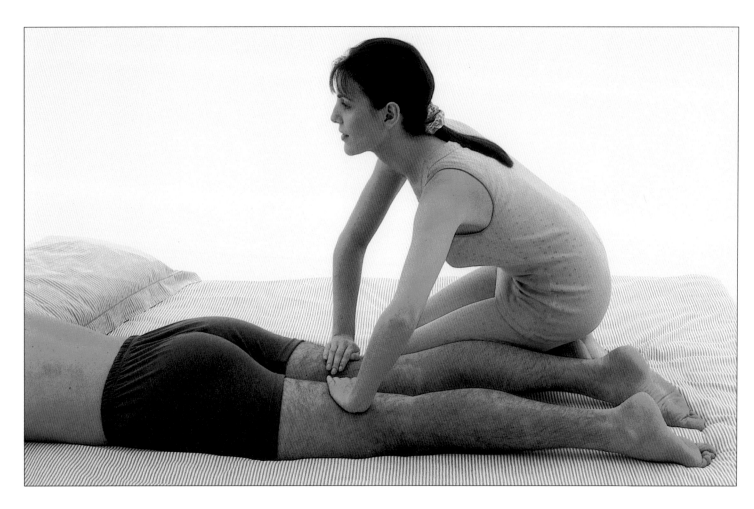

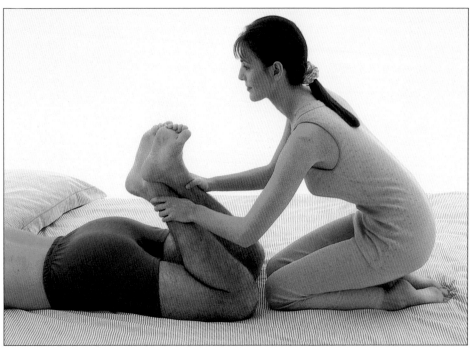

1 ▲ Start by stroking to feel any tense areas or tight muscles. Sit or kneel by the side of the sufferer's legs and move up as you stroke. Place your hands, palms down, over each ankle, with your fingers across the calf and pointing inwards. Press and slide your hands all the way up the legs in one smooth, firm, fast stroke to the top of the thighs. Repeat up to 20 times.

2 ◀ Cross his feet at the heels, pick them up and slowly bend them up and back towards his bottom until you meet resistance. Hold the stretch for a count of 15, then release and repeat. Then do a slow friction rub over calves and thighs: place your hands, palms down, across the leg and rub them backwards and forwards in a sawing motion.

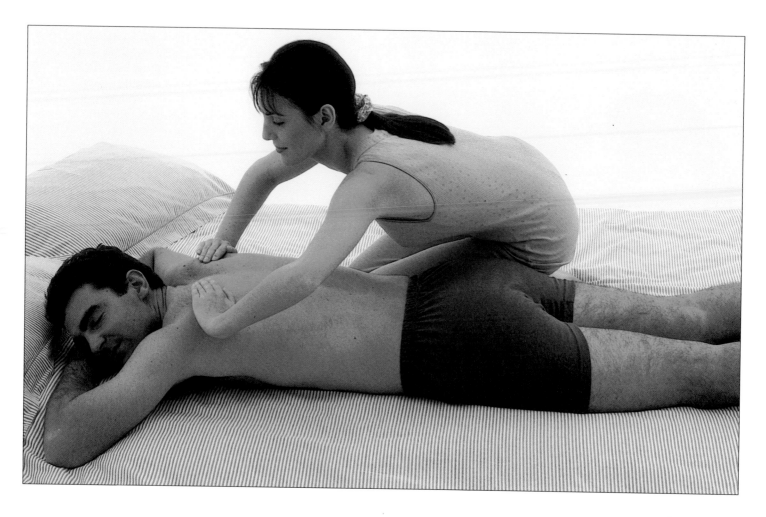

3 ▲ Kneel by the sufferer's hip, covering the lower body if necessary to keep it warm. Do one firm stroke all the way up the back, fanning your hands out at the top of the shoulders and turning them to pull down the arms to feel any tense areas. Start with your palms down, hands on the lower back with fingers pointing into the spine. Repeat up to 20 times, as a slow, firm, flowing stroke.

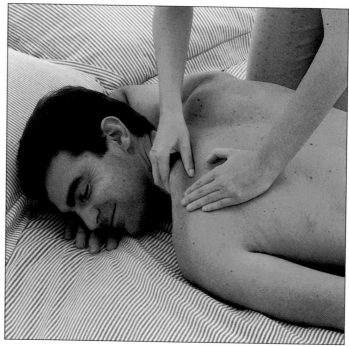

4 ▶ Now go back to any tense or knotted areas on the back and deep knead them by picking up and squeezing the flesh between the fingers and thumb of each hand. Spend quite a lot of time across the tops of the shoulders and the lower back. Make small circular strokes with your thumbs alone under the shoulder blades and up the nape of the neck.

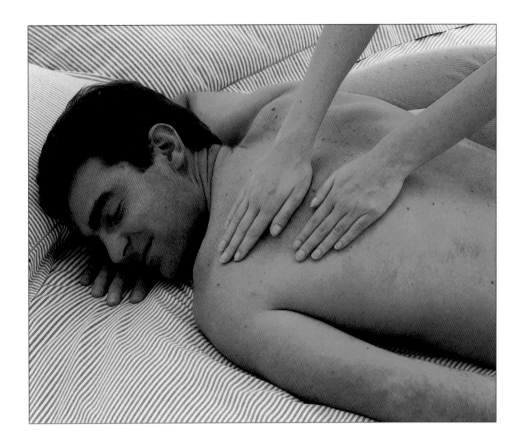

5 ◀ Do a fast, sweeping friction rub with your hands palms down and moving vigorously so each stroke is about 20 cm (8 inches) long. Keeping your hands parallel, rub up and down from the lower back to the shoulder tops on either side of the spine. Keep it going for several minutes, getting slower towards the end, but still rubbing firmly.

6 ▶ The person being massaged should turn over so that he is lying face up. Cover the upper body to keep it warm. Hold one foot around the top of the instep, prop it against your knee or thigh and flex backwards by gently pushing up the toes. Hold for a count of five, then release. In the same position, move the toes from side to side and make slow circles with them in the air. Then place the palm of each hand on the top of the thighs and stroke slowly and firmly down to the toes in one movement. Repeat several times. Finally, hold the feet under the heels and round the back of the ankle, take their weight and gently pull the legs away from the body. Hold for a count of ten, then repeat.

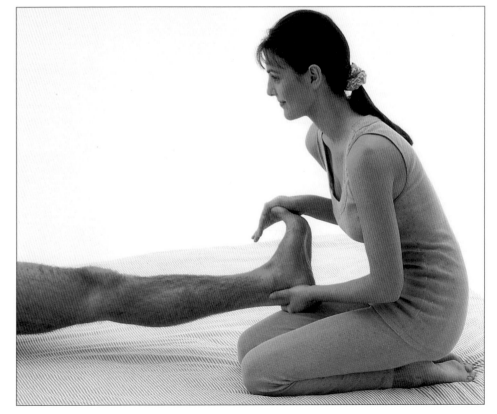

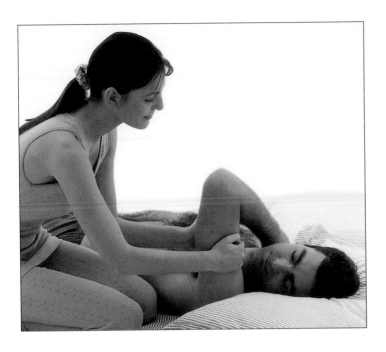

7 ◄ Hold the sufferer's hand, palm to palm, and interlock your fingers, pushing his hand gently back and forwards to flex and stretch it. Then place the palms of your hands around his upper arm and lift it, letting his elbow bend and the hand relax down to the chest. Then push in and squeeze with the heels and palms of your hands all the way down the arm to the wrist, avoiding the bony elbow. Finish off by placing your hands, palms down, around the top of the arm and sliding them both right down the arm to the wrist, holding the hand and gently pulling it away from the body. Repeat on the other arm.

8 ► Kneeling or sitting by the sufferer's head, turn it to one side and use one hand, palm down, followed by the other, to stroke across the shoulder, up the side of the neck, over the jaw and cheek, to the temple, forehead and through the scalp to the crown of the head. As you reach the face, lift your palm so that you use fingers only to continue the stroke up into the hair. Work on only one side at a time for up to 20 strokes, getting slower and gentler to the end. Gently lift and turn the head to the other side and repeat the entire step again on the other half of

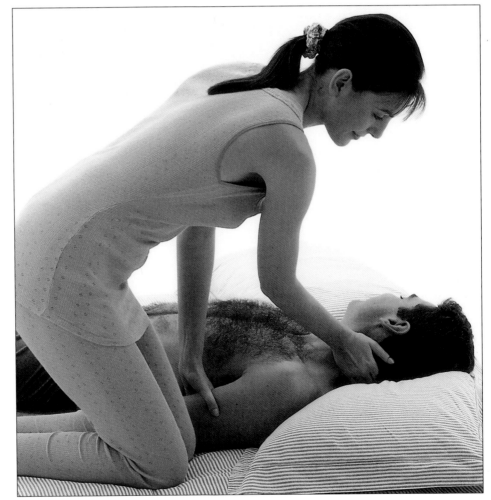

81

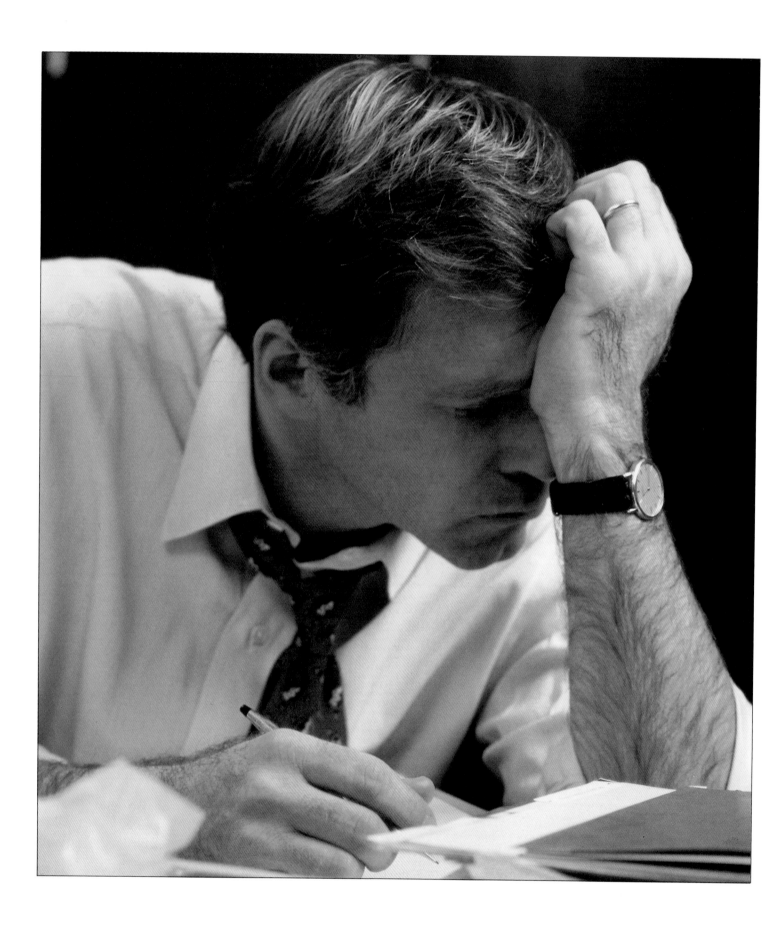

MASSAGE FOR THE 'MORNING AFTER'

✻

It does not matter whether you wake up jetlagged or with a hangover, the worst thing about the 'morning after' is that it takes all the pleasure out of the night before. Too much time in the air or too much alcohol leave you with similar symptoms – dazed, glassy-eyed, dehydrated, bloated, dry-mouthed, headachy, unable to concentrate, sometimes even unable to finish a sentence.

Everybody seems to have a pet cure for a hangover, ranging from eating a raw egg to a three-course meal, or from drinking strong coffee to drinking more alcohol. Similarly, frequent travellers try everything from turning their clocks forward before they get on the plane to taking a sleeping tablet as soon as they get off. However, the only things that really do help cure that morning after misery are getting as much sleep and drinking as much water as possible.

While you wait for nature to take its course, this soothing massage will help get rid of the headache and, if you have not fallen asleep by the end, it will leave you in better condition to cope with the demands of the day. It is a simple series of gentle presses and slow, relaxing strokes to the nape of the neck, forehead, temples, eyes and scalp – and these are the areas that jetlag and a hangover seem to hit worse.

HOW TO DO THE 'MORNING AFTER' MASSAGE

To make the massage even more soothing, put some ice in a plastic bag and roll it in a towel to slip under the back of the sufferer's neck as a therapeutic pillow. Dip cotton wool pads in iced water or milk, squeeze them out and place them over the eyes. Keep the room warm and dimly lit and make sure that the person you are going to massage is lying, stretched out and as comfortable as possible, especially if he hopes to go to sleep.

The good thing about this massage is that you can do it anywhere. The movements are so simple that you do not need oil, and you can adapt the steps and do them while the sufferer is fully clothed and sitting upright in a low chair at work, if need be. Remember that the secret of its success is to do all strokes slowly, soothingly and repeatedly, as if you were trying to pacify a fractious baby – and then, it works!

(Left) Jetlag or a hangover can turn a normal day's work into an agonizing ordeal.

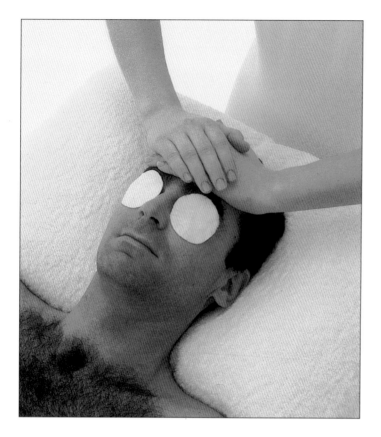

1 ◄ Start with a series of head presses. Cup your hands, palms down, over the forehead. Gently press down for a count of ten, relax for a count of five and then repeat. Push the lower hand backwards with the upper hand in a firm forehead stroke. Then place hands, palms down, on the sides of the head from the crown down to the ears. Press firmly in for a count of ten, relax for five, then repeat. Slide your hands, palms up, under the nape of the neck, then gently lift to stretch the neck without raising the head. Hold for a count of ten, then relax.

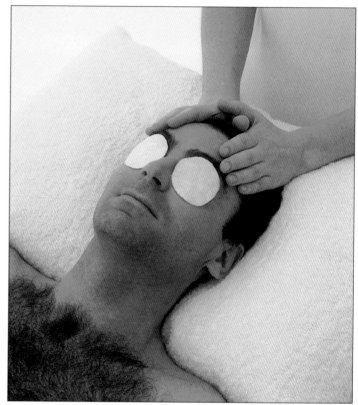

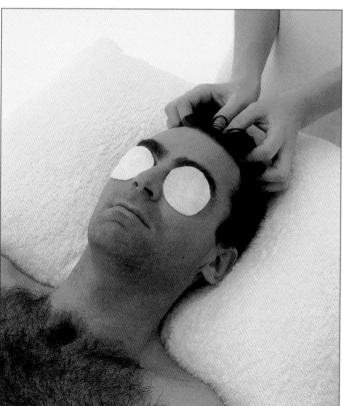

2 ▲ Now massage the forehead. Stroke firmly upward with the fingers of each hand, one after the other, starting between the brows and pulling back to the hairline. Every sixth stroke, slide the fingers out to follow the contours of each brow and end by gently pressing in with your fingertips over the temples. Finish off by using the palm of one hand, followed by the other, rhythmically stroking from the brow right up to the crown of the head for several minutes.

3 ◄ Bend your fingers into stiff claws and rake the scalp from the hairline up to the crown all over the head, including the nape of the neck. Repeat for several minutes, then gently press into the head all around the hairline with stiff fingertips and make circles on the scalp. Next, hold small sections of hair close to the roots and gently tug, repeating all over the head. Finish off with long, slow finger strokes through the scalp that end by gently pulling the hair away from the head.

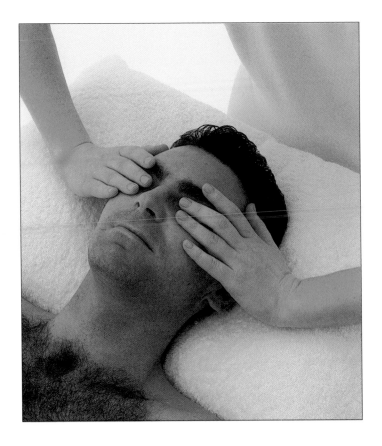

4 ◄ Start with your palms across the forehead, fingertips touching above the nose. All movements should be gentle. Slowly slide your hands down until the middle and ring fingers are resting lightly over the eyes. Press in, holding for a count of eight, then lightly slide fingers out across the eyes to the temples. Press in over each temple with the first two fingers of each hand and make circles to rotate the skin. Then repeat several times. Finally, place an index fingertip over each tear duct and lightly press into the eye corner. Hold for a count of five, then release.

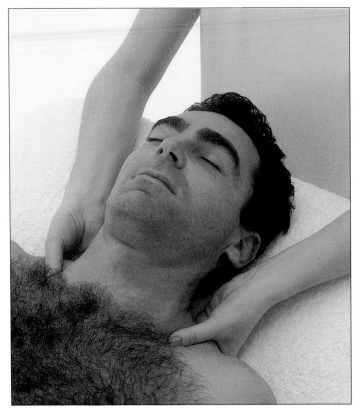

5 ▲ Knead the top of the shoulder muscle, starting close to the neck and work out towards the arm. After several minutes, place the palm of one hand over the top of the arm and pull up, in one smooth stroke, along the shoulder and neck to the ear. As one hand gets to the end of the stroke, the other should be starting the next one. Then repeat all of step five on the other shoulder muscle.

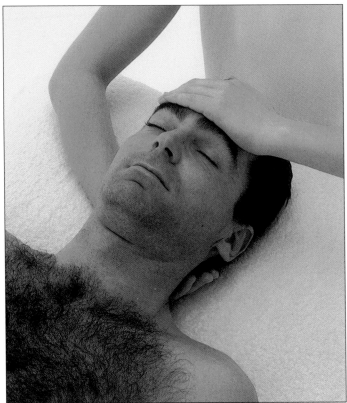

6 ◄ Now place your right hand, palm up, under the top of the neck, with your thumb to one ear and fingers to the other. Gently knead and press inwards along the base of the skull bone and the top of the vertebrae. With your right hand in the same position, place your left hand, palm down, across the forehead and gently press downwards as you lift up with your right hand. Hold for a count of five, then relax. Finish off with soothing forehead strokes, one hand following the other, getting slower and slower until you stop.

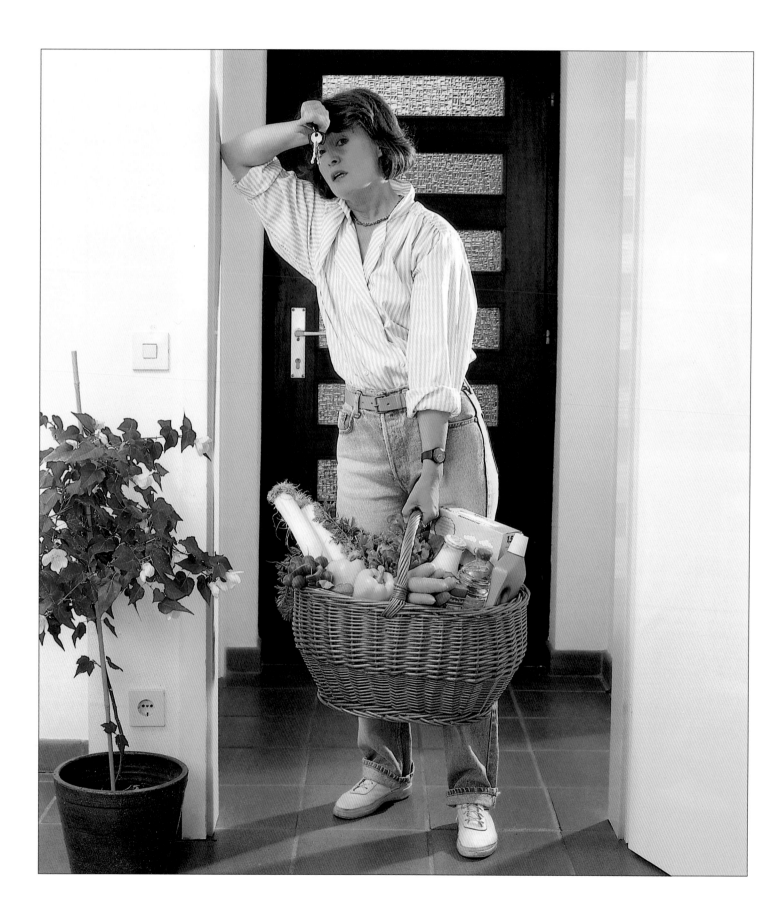

MASSAGE FOR BACK ACHE

✳

At some point in their lives, three out of four people will have problems with their backs. The commonest triggers are lifting a heavy weight (pregnancy, carrying a washing machine up a flight of stairs), a sudden jerky movement (a sneeze, throwing a punch), or just regularly resisting the pull of gravity (standing all day, sitting over a word processor). Once the initial damage is done, almost anything – including stress – can make the muscles seize up and bring on the agony.

Fortunately, the back is not only the easiest part of the body to massage, being such a large, smooth area, but it also responds instantly to being rubbed the right way. Remember that the spine carries nerve fibres that affect the entire body and so the pleasure of a back massage spreads from top to toe. The back also has more muscles than any other part of the body and does most of the work of keeping us upright throughout our waking hours. So it needs all the help it can get.

When using massage to relieve any kind of back pain, feel your way slowly, be gentle and use light, rhythmic strokes. Always consult your doctor before having back massage if you have had surgery or are currently undergoing treatment for any kind of back complaint.

How to Massage the Back

The best position for having a back massage is lying face down. It is important that the person being massaged is comfortable, so he should lie on a well-padded floor or firm mattress. Place a rolled towel or small pillow under the upper chest and neck so that the head can relax in the face-down position and not twist to one side, which can cause strain.

Cover any areas not being worked on with towels to keep them warm. Make sure the massage oil is handy before beginning. Here are two back massages shown step-by-step: the first concentrates on the lower back, the second (see page 90) on the upper back. However, the two combine quite naturally for an all-over therapeutic and relaxing routine.

(Left) Back pain may mean that simply picking up a shopping bag results in weeks of agony.

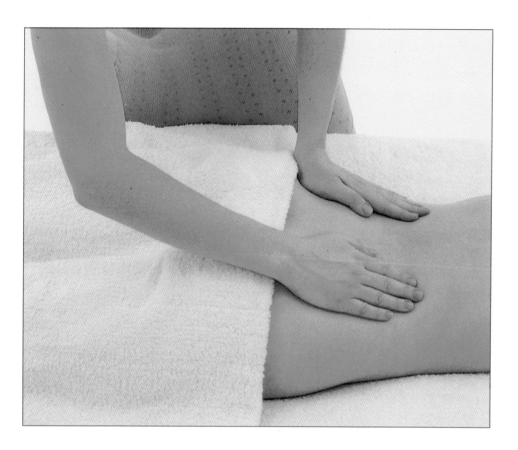

MASSAGE FOR LOWER BACK ACHE

1 ◄ Remember that all strokes should be slow, light, gentle and rhythmic, with lots of repetitions. Stand or kneel at the top of the thigh throughout. Start with your palms down on either side of the base of the spine (the tailbone or sacrum) about 5 cm (2 inches) away from the spine. Gently slide your hands up to the waist, fan them out to each side and pull down the sides of the torso, then back across the buttocks to the start position. Keep repeating the stroke without pausing. The upward movement is light, but the out and downward may be firmer.

2 ▶ Next, place palms down, with one hand on top of the other. Make slow, gentle circles all over the buttocks and lower back muscles from waist to tailbone. Keep your fingers flat, but relaxed, so that the light pressure comes from the heel and palm of the hand as you make circles, rather than from the fingers. Do not massage directly over the spine at any time – keep the circle movements on either side of the vertebrae all around the lower back. This stroke should be gentle and continuous so that it is warming and relaxing.

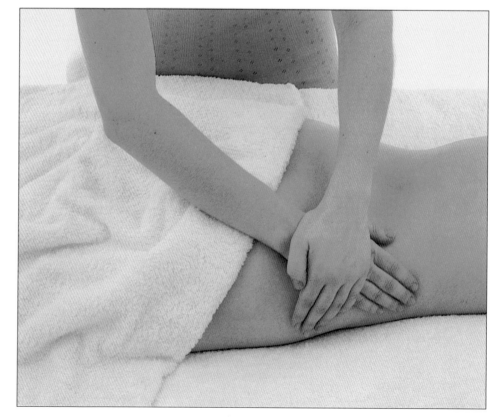

3 ▶ Now do a gentle, light-pressure thumbing stroke. Place each thumb on either side of the spine about 5 cm (2 inches) away from it. Make small circles, with the thumbs working together so that one makes clockwise circles while the other moves anti-clockwise. Gradually move from the base of the tailbone up to the waist, keeping your thumbs to the side of the spine, never directly on it. Repeat the stroke, working further out towards the hips each time. Keep the stroke light, but it can be firmer over areas of knotted muscle as long as they are not tender or sore.

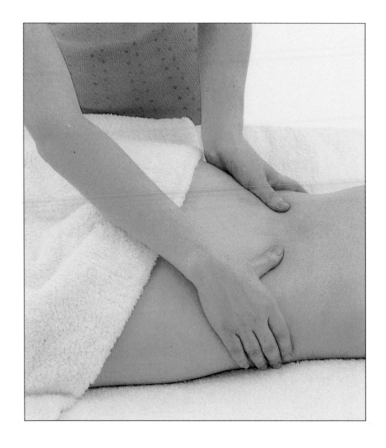

4 ▼ Stand or kneel at one side and, reaching across the lower back, tuck the fingers of one hand, palm down, under the top of the thigh. Using firm fingers, pull the flesh back up towards the spine. As the first hand pulls upwards, tuck the other hand into the start position and repeat the movement, so one hand follows the other in a smooth, stroking motion. Make sure the firm upwards pull lasts the length of the stroke from the side of the torso into the middle of the back. Work up both sides from hip to waist.

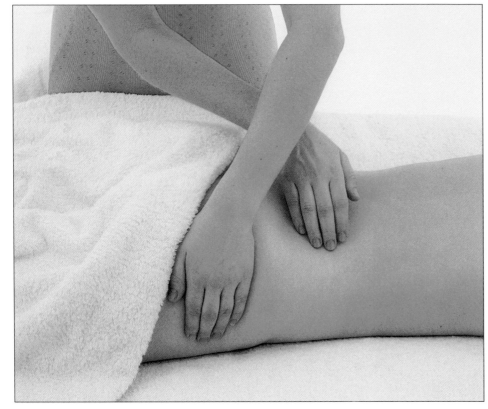

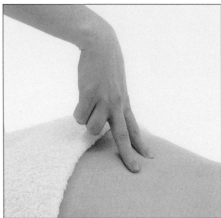

5 ▲ Place the first two fingers of one hand stiffly 5 cm (2 inches) apart on either side of the spine at the nape of the neck. Run them gently, slowly, with an even pressure, from the neck down to the tailbone. Repeat several times. Finish off by repeating step 1 again, or any of the steps that were particularly soothing to the back ache. If any of the strokes causes discomfort, stop immediately – this massage is for pleasure, not pain.

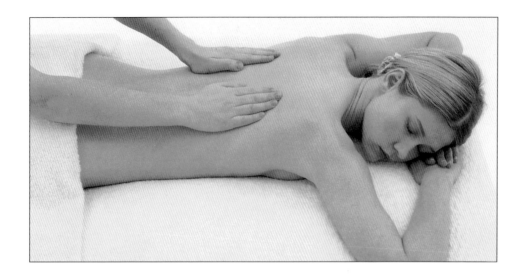

MASSAGE FOR UPPER BACK ACHE

1 ◀ Remember that all strokes should be slow, light, gentle and rhythmic, with lots of repetitions. Stand or kneel at the side throughout. Start with your palms down on either side of the lower spine about 5 cm (2 inches) away from it. Gently slide your hands up over the waist to the shoulders, fan them out to each side and pull down the sides of the torso across the hips to the start position. Keep repeating the stroke without pausing. The upward movement is light, but the out and downward may be firmer to stretch and pull flesh.

2 ▶ Using your thumb and fingers in a light pinching movement and working with both hands together, knead the soft tissue from the waist all up the back, paying particular attention to any tight or knotty areas around the tops of the shoulders. Do not knead on any bony parts, avoid the spine and do not pinch in too deeply if it causes discomfort – a light, plucking movement is just as relaxing on tender muscles as firmer pressure. Keep kneading rhythmically for several minutes as this will help warm and relax any tense, tight places.

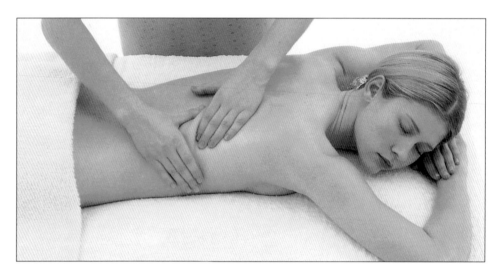

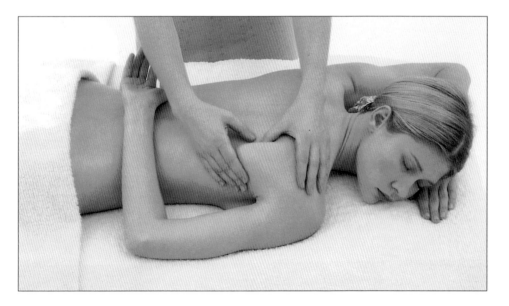

3 ◀ To release tension in the shoulders and relax the upper back, bend the arm of the person being massaged at the elbow and place the hand, palm up, on the lower back – this will make the shoulder bone jut out so that you can massage the muscles underneath it. Rest the elbow on your knee, so that it does not flop down, and bend over to knead, using thumbs only, under and around the projecting shoulder blade. Knead using deep, flicking, rhythmic thumb movements, followed by small thumb circles and finish with long, slow strokes the length of the shoulder blade using the sides of the thumbs.

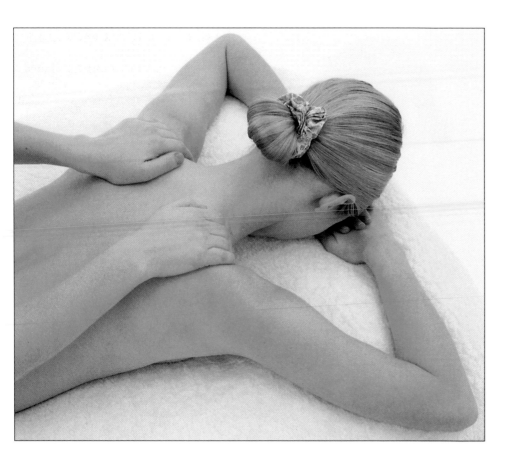

4 ◀ Concentrate on the muscles that run across the top of the shoulders. Place your hands, palms down, on either side of the neck so that the fingers curve over the top of the shoulders and rest on the collar bone. Pull the flesh firmly back, one hand after the other in a rhythmic stroke, keeping your fingers stiff and using an inward pressure to pull and stretch the muscles. It should be a continuous, flowing movement. Then use both hands to squeeze and knead each shoulder muscle from the arm across to the neck on each side.

5 ▶ To loosen the back, hold the top of each arm and gently pull the shoulders back until they are slightly raised. Hold for a count of ten, then lower and repeat. Next, place relaxed hands, palms down, over the spine in the middle of the back. Glide hands apart diagonally, so one goes to the hip and the other to the opposite shoulder. Do not press down, but pull crosswise to stretch the skin and muscles. Hold for a count of ten, then repeat on the other side. If any of the steps or strokes in this massage cause discomfort, stop immediately.

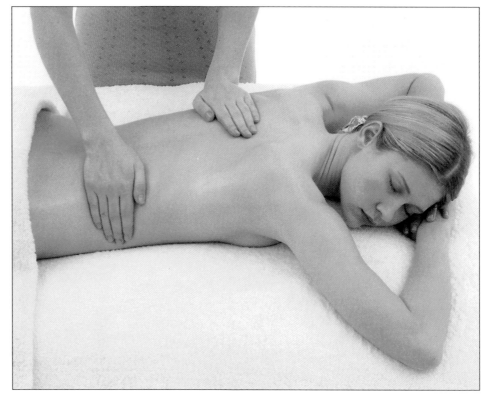

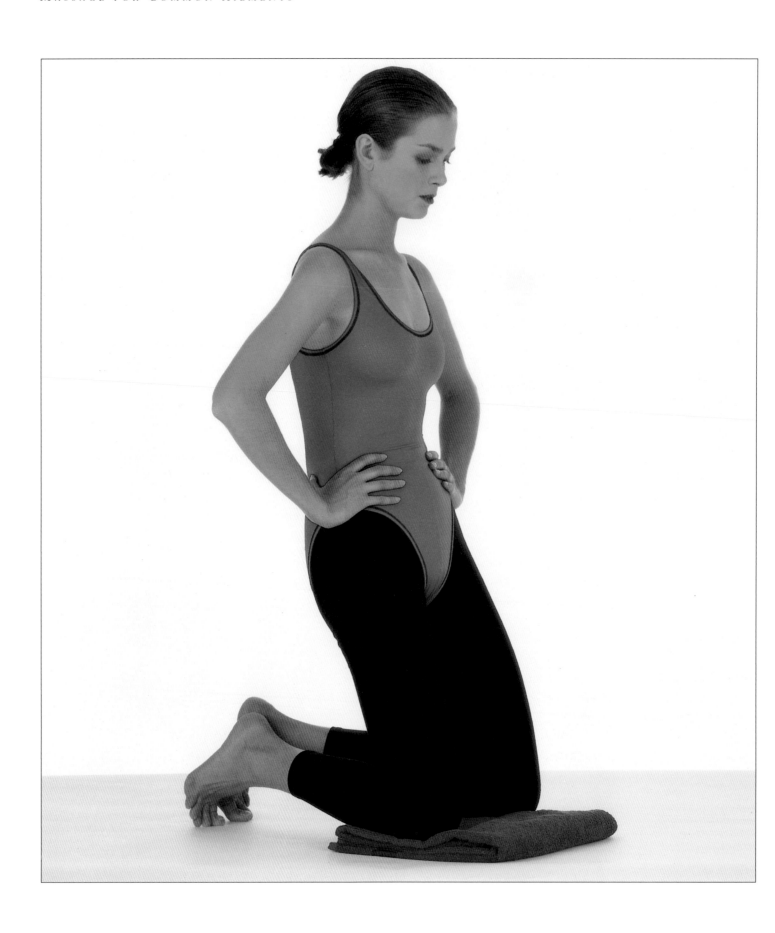

MASSAGE FOR SORE MUSCLES

Muscles ache for all sorts of reasons. Tension or bad posture can make them ache, running a race or carrying a heavy load can make them sore and a sprain or sudden jerk can cause agony. However, once again, massage works miracles with any kind of sore muscles, as it not only soothes them but, in most cases, it also manages to heal them.

The most frequent muscular aches are usually caused by a build up of lactic acid, which occurs when muscles are exercised so vigorously that body wastes are trapped within them. This happens to athletes all the time. Research into sports medicine has proved that muscles recover five times faster if they are rubbed rather than rested in between bouts of energetic exercise. This is the reason why you see athletes being massaged, from Olympic level down to the local team.

To get the same benefits at home, you must massage sore muscles with firm or fast rhythmic strokes, to warm and relax them, then do some stretches to keep them loose. This massage concentrates on the largest muscle groups – calves, thighs, buttocks, biceps, shoulders and back. So do as many repeats as possible of strokes that go over areas of soreness, and fewer or none of the others.

However, never take any of the stretches farther than is comfortable and keep friction rubs or kneading strokes light over any areas that are very sore. If the aching has not gone from muscles after two days, seek medical advice as they may be injured rather than just over-exerted.

HOW TO MASSAGE SORE MUSCLES

Try to make all strokes rhythmic and repetitive so that they are as warming as possible. It helps if you rub in some liniment or eucalyptus essential oil, as well as your massage oil; the menthol heats skin and soothes muscles even more. If you have a warm bath beforehand, the sore muscles will respond better to the massage and hurt less.

If muscles are stiff as well as sore, it is more comfortable to have a pillow under the knees (to relax leg and back muscles) for the first half of the massage.

(Left) Even gentle forms of exercise can cause aches which benefit from massage.

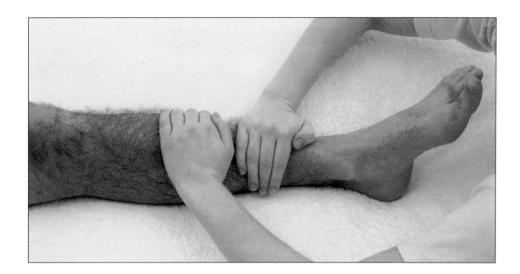

1 ◁ Place your hands, palms down, across the left leg, with fingers pointing in opposite directions. Then gently push down and slide your hands up from the ankle to knee. Move your hands over the knee lightly, then continue the stroke with downward pressure up to the thigh. Slide your hands back down along the sides of the leg and repeat for several minutes. Then do a fast, firm friction rub, with palms flat, from feet up to the thighs.

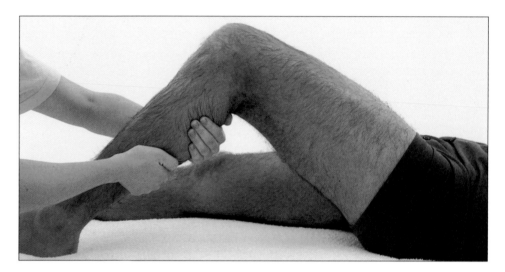

2 ▷ Bend the left leg up at the knee and prop the foot against your thigh for support. Place your hands, palms up, around the back of the calf muscle above the ankle. Wring the leg by sliding your hands backwards and forwards in opposite directions to twist the flesh. Keep the motion going and gradually work up the back of the leg from ankle to knee. Repeat two or three times.

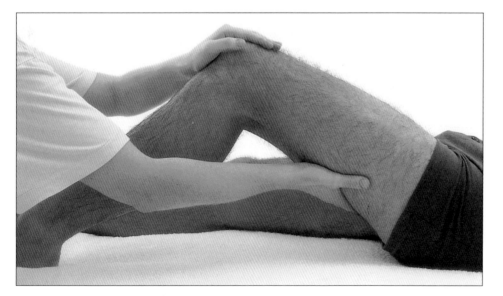

3 ◁ In the same position, knead and stroke the back of the thigh. Place your right hand, palm up, behind the knee, with your thumb on the outer thigh and your fingers to the inner side so that your hand makes a V shape. Press and pinch in as you push the hand up the leg to the top of the thigh, to give a deep, kneading stroke. Bring the fingers together, slide round to the front of the thigh and back down to the knee. Then repeat for several minutes.

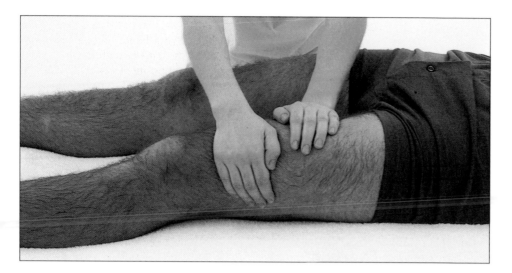

4 ◄ With the left leg straight again, start a criss-cross stroke from the ankle to thigh. Place your hands, palms down, across the leg with your fingers pointing to the inner ankle. Then do a firm stroke from one side of the leg to the other, so that your hands criss-cross and one pushes forward as the other pulls backwards. Make sure your fingers curve under the leg on the downward inner stroke and that the heels of your hands push into the outer leg on the upward stroke.

5 ► Now the person being massaged should bend the left leg and keep the other straight while you stand at his feet. Bend forward from the waist and pick up the bent leg, placing the heel on your shoulder. Keep your own legs apart with your knees slightly bent to avoid straining your back, then gently place one hand behind the knee and one behind the ankle for support, and straighten the leg as you push up slightly with your shoulder. Hold this stretch for a count of 15, then release your hands so the knee relaxes. Now do steps one to five on the other leg.

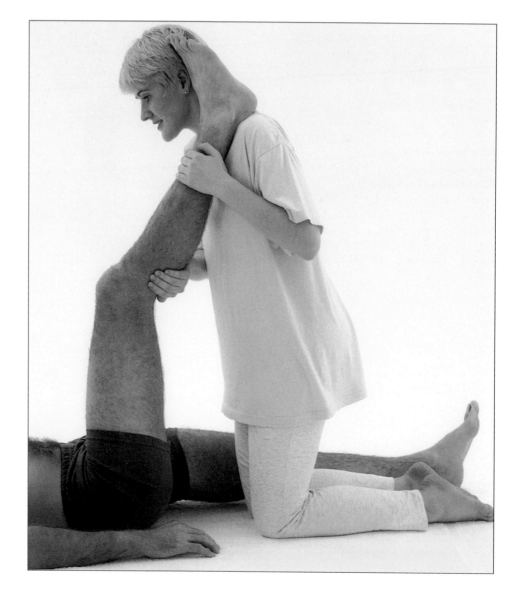

6 ▶ Place your hands palm down over the upper arm and biceps. Do a fast, firm friction rub so that your hands make a sawing motion. Place your palms down around the wrist, with fingers pointing in opposite directions. Slide your hands up the arm, moving together in a slow, firm stroke from wrist to shoulder, but being gentle over the elbow joint. From the shoulder, slowly pull your hands down the sides of the arm. Repeat for several minutes.

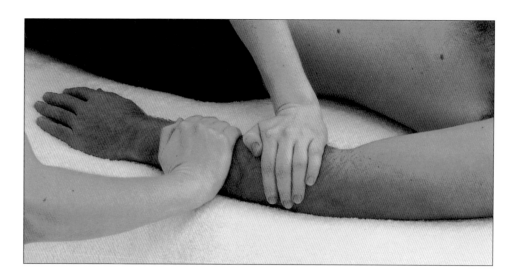

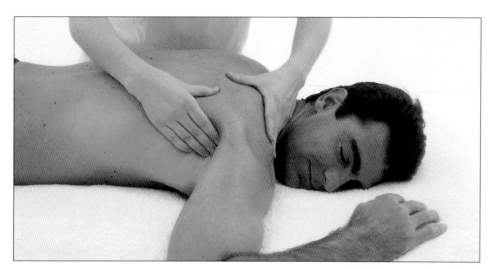

7 ◀ The person being massaged should turn over to lie face down. Knead the muscles, pinching the flesh between your thumbs and fingers, right across the shoulders, upper arms and middle of the back. Then do a firm, flat-handed stroke from below the shoulder blade diagonally up to the opposite shoulder, repeating several times on both sides. Finish with a firm, fast friction rub from the middle of the back up and over the

8 ▶ Make your hands into loose fists and pummel all over the upper back, using the base of the fist in an up-and-down hammer movement, one hand after the other. Keep your fists relaxed so that your hands bounce off the body and avoid the spine and bony shoulder blades. Then pummel the buttock muscles between hips and thighs, using the same fist movement. Finish by doing firm palm strokes in circles over the buttocks and the top of the back.

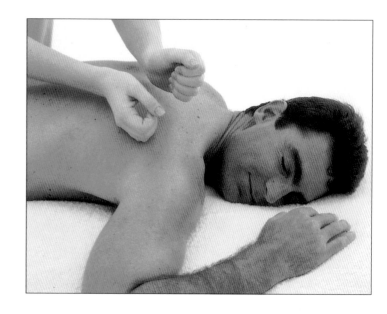

9 ▶ With your hands, palms down, between the shoulder blades, press down and slide your hands diagonally out to the tops of the arms, then pull them in across the shoulder tops and up the sides of the neck, before sliding them lightly back down either side of the spine to the start position. Next, with palms down below one shoulder blade, glide them upward in a diagonal direction to the top of the arm, fan them out in a circle and draw them together at the start. Repeat as a smooth, flowing stroke.

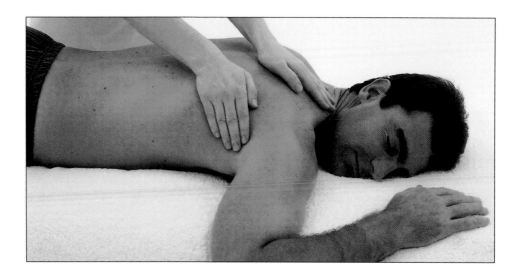

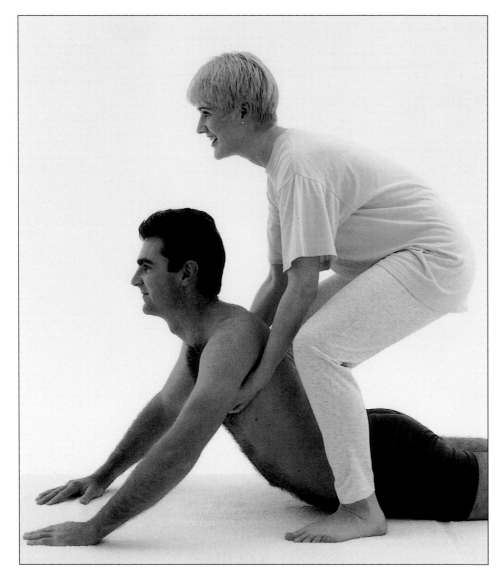

10 ◀ Please take special note of lifting instructions for this massage. To stretch and release tension in the lower back and shoulder muscles, do a half-body lift. Stand astride the hips of the person being massaged and slide your hands under his arms to the front of his chest. Gently and slowly pull the torso upwards, bending your knees to take the strain off your back, and stretch him up as far as is comfortable. Hold for a count of 15, then relax back down. Repeat twice more.

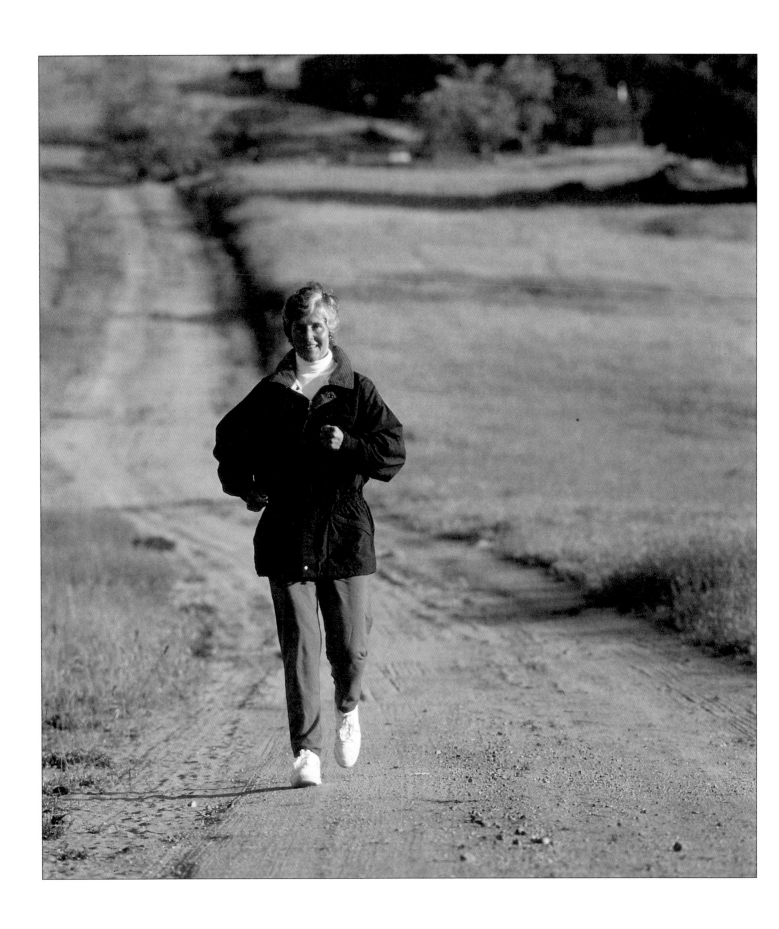

MASSAGE FOR SORE FEET

Nearly 200,000 years ago, people first stood up on two feet and walked.
Since then, those feet have kept on walking and are largely ignored by modern man
and woman. Most of us tend to notice them only when something goes
wrong – a callus, a corn, aches, blisters or bunions usually
get attention, but not the feet themselves.

They get stuffed into shoes that rub or socks that make them sweat. They have to
totter on too-high heels or be squeezed, toes-first, into pointy tipped shoes.
They must run and jump and kick and climb and carry us and all our baggage
everywhere we want to go. Not only are feet ignored and taken for granted,
but nearly everyone thinks they are ugly or smelly.

However, the truth of the matter is that feet can give more pleasure than many of the
body's more glamorous zones. Almost every nerve ending in the body –
and there are about 72,000 of them – finishes up in each foot, tangled around a
web of 38 muscles and 28 tiny bones. This is why feet are so strong but sensitive.
If you massage them, you send waves of pleasure from toe to top and can relax the
entire body. A good foot massage can get rid of aches, help keep feet flexible,
healthy and happy, lighten your step and improve your mood.

HOW TO MASSAGE SORE FEET

If your feet constantly ache or hurt, you should buy new shoes, see a chiropodist and
have them massaged at the end of every day. This foot massage is most enjoyable
if it is given while you lie on your back and relax. However, life is too cruel to let us
have total enjoyment, so you can easily adapt it to do as a self-massage if you must.
To do it yourself, sit comfortably and rest the ankle of the foot you are working on
across the knee of the other leg, then follow the eight steps in the same way.

You will need lots of oil, as feet have naturally dry, thick skin. Work gently on the top
of the foot because the bones are close to the surface here, but be firmer on the sole.
If feet are ticklish, try making all movements slower and deeper. However,
some people's feet are so sensitive that massage is impossible.

(Left) There is nothing so enjoyable as a foot massage after a long walk.

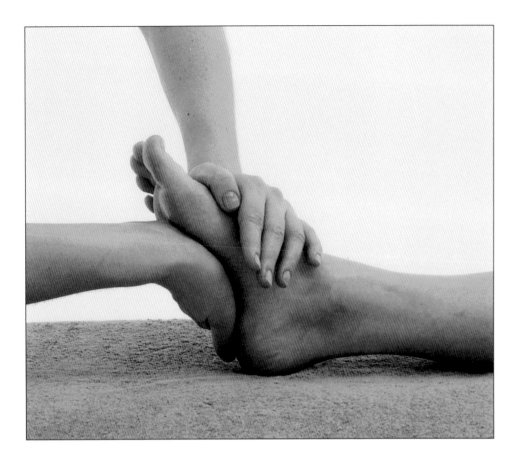

1 ◄ Do all the steps on one foot and then on the other. Start with a friction rub. Sandwich the entire foot between the palms of your hands and rub briskly so that one hand goes forward as the other moves back. Use lots of oil to warm and relax the foot. To do the heel, lift the foot up and prop it across your leg. Place your hands parallel to the calf, then rub up and down.

2 ▶ Do a series of long, slow strokes pulling from the ankle to toes. Place one hand on the back of the heel and the other over the front of the ankle to sandwich the foot between your palms. Pull firmly and press in as you glide your hands back to the toes, following the contours of the foot throughout. Repeat as a smooth, flowing stroke for several minutes.

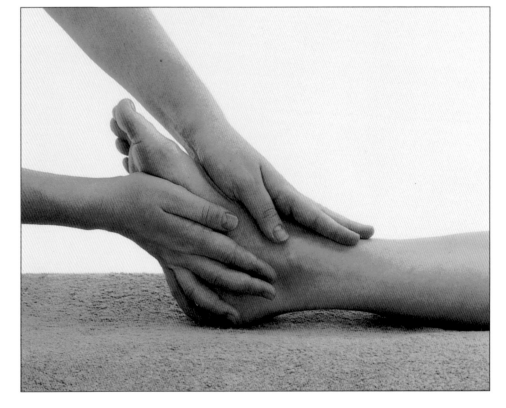

3 ▶ Stretch the foot by flexing upwards. Lift the foot by holding with the left hand behind the ankle. Place the palm of your right hand flat against the sole of the foot and push in to follow the contours closely, then gently push against the toes of the foot to flex back up towards the leg. Hold for a count of ten, then relax and repeat four times.

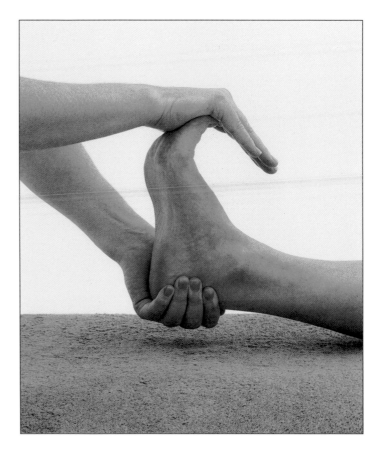

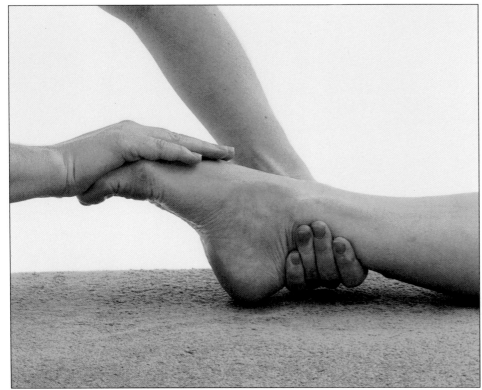

4 ◀ Stretch the foot by flexing downwards. Place the palm of your left hand around the ankle to support the foot. Then wrap the right palm over the toes, with your thumb under the sole of the foot. Gently push the toes downwards, hold for a count of ten, then relax and repeat four times. In the same position, gently push the foot from side to side five times.

5 ▶ Wrap your fingers around the top of the foot and use your thumbs to make small circles all over the sole of the foot from under the toes back to the heel. Then, keeping your thumbs stiff, use them to push and stroke, with one thumb following the other, all over the sole of the foot from the heel back up to the toes.

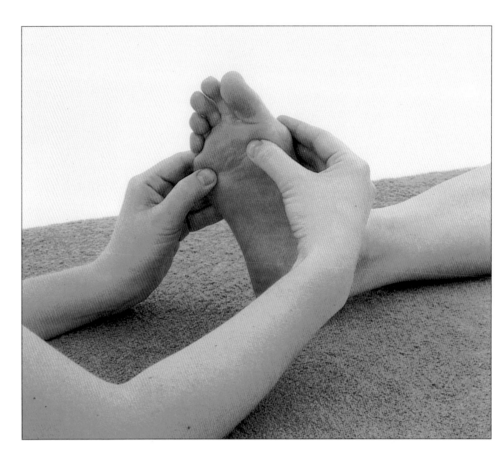

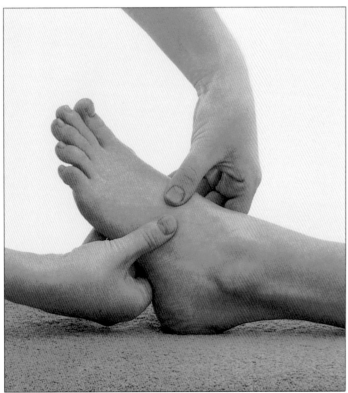

6 ◀ Wrap your fingers under the arch of the foot with your thumbs on the instep at the front. Use your thumbs to make small circles all over the top of the foot and all around the ankle bone. Then, keeping your thumbs stiff, use them lightly to stroke all over the top of the foot from the toes back up to the ankle, with one following the other.

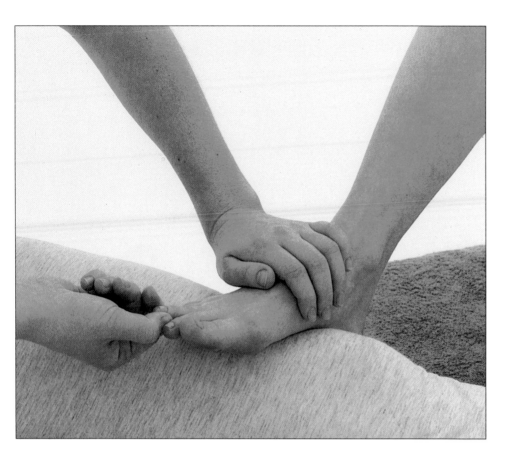

7 ◄ Next massage the toes. Hold the foot firmly around the arch with your left hand; take the foot off the ground and rest it on your bent knee or thigh. Then do three different strokes on each toe: a rub, a pull and a twist. Hold each toe between your right hand thumb and index finger, using lots of oil, and working from the foot up towards the tip of the toe.

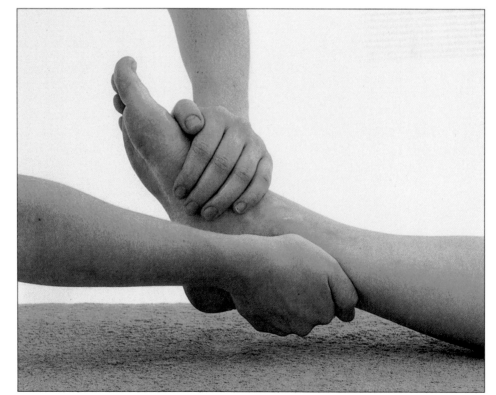

8 ► Place your right hand, palm up, against the back of the ankle and, wrapping your fingers to one side and your thumb to the other, squeeze into the tendon behind the ankle bone to hold the foot firmly. With the left hand, palm down across the instep, firmly stroke the top of the foot from ankle to toes in a flowing movement, getting slower and lighter till you stop.

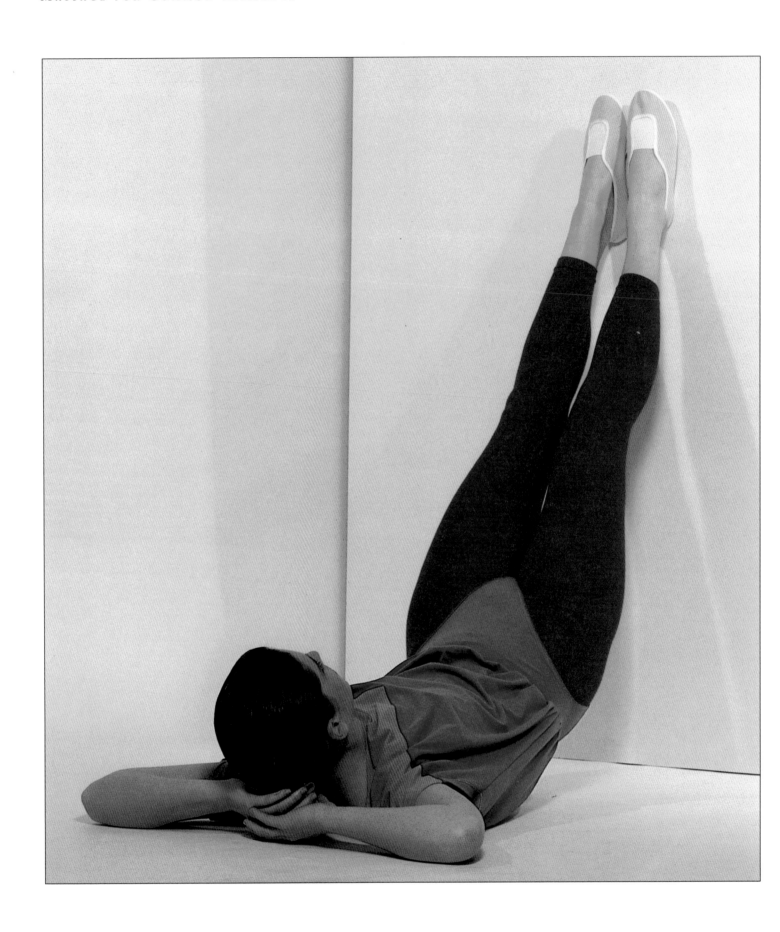

MASSAGE FOR TIRED AND ACHING LEGS

In a single stride, you use more than 100 different muscles. These same muscles have to carry twice your body weight with the impact of every step you take. Even if you stand as still as a stork all day, they take the strain and support you so that you do not fall over. In addition, it is these same muscles that let you do fancy steps as you dodge the traffic or dance the night away.

The legs take this kind of physical abuse in their stride, since a trip, run, hop and jump are all in a day's work. However, after a long day they get tired and affect the whole body, so you shuffle around in a bad mood rather than tripping about with a smile and a skip. This is the time for a massage, as it will not only relax your legs, but also recharge flagging energy levels enough for them to carry you through a night on the town.

However, if you push it too far – either by over-exercising or standing for long periods day after day – the leg muscles really do rebel and they ache, stiffen, swell and knot with pain, which can cause long-term leg problems, such as varicose veins or oedema. So if you over-exercise frequently, if you stand for long periods every day, if you are pregnant or very overweight, you should have regular leg massages as a preventative measure to help relax the muscles and boost the blood circulation.

HOW TO MASSAGE TIRED OR ACHING LEGS

For the greatest benefit, you need firm upward massage strokes and fast friction rubs to relax the large leg muscles and help the blood flow back up against the pull of gravity. As the legs have few natural oil-producing sebaceous glands, use lots of oil to keep the skin soft and supple all year round.

A leg massage is most comfortable for someone lying down on a firm surface. If he is on the floor, you will have to kneel to massage him; otherwise, he should be lying high enough for you to stand comfortably so you that you do not strain your back. While you work on one leg, cover the other with towels to keep it warm. After the massage, he should lie down for ten minutes with feet propped up on pillows or against a wall, so they are higher than the head.

(Left) Look after your leg muscles, and they will respond with renewed energy.

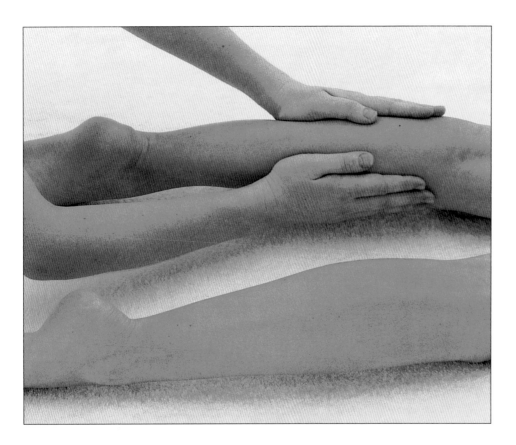

1 ◀ For steps one to five, the person being massaged should lie face down. Starting at the feet, stroke up the sides of the left leg from ankle to thigh. Place each hand, palms down, just above the ankle bone, with your fingers together pointing forwards. As you push up the leg, press in firmly with the heel of your hands and keep your fingers relaxed. Release the pressure as you glide your hands over the knee joint, then press in again to the thigh top. On the downward stroke, keep the movement gentle, using your fingers lightly to stretch the skin back towards the foot.

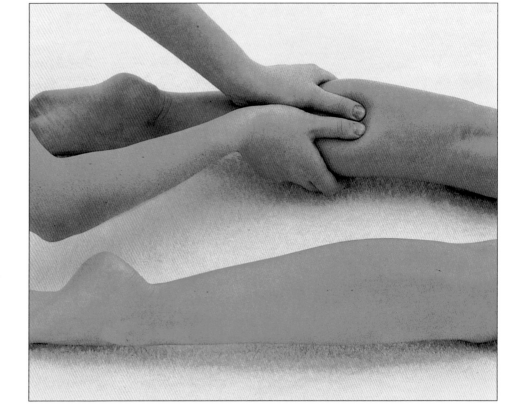

2 ▶ Stretch the back of the left leg by gently bending the heel up towards the bottom as far as is comfortable. Hold for a count of five, then relax and repeat. Place your thumbs together on the outer leg above the ankle bone. Press in with your thumbs and slowly slide them upwards along the calf muscle to the knee. Repeat, working in lines upwards so that you thumb-stroke the entire calf from outer across to inner leg.

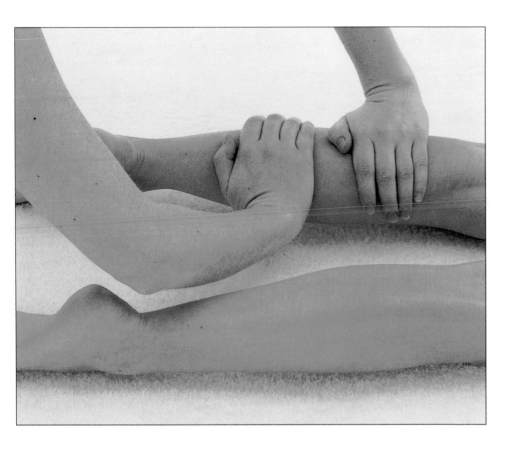

3 ◀ Now work from the upper calf up to the top of the thigh on the left leg. Place your hands, palms down, positioned across the leg so that your fingers are pointing in opposite directions. With a firm downward pressure, slide both hands upwards in one long stroke from the knee to the thigh top. Fan your hands out in opposite directions at the top of the thigh and draw each hand back down the side of the leg to the knee. It is a firm upwards pressure and a lighter downward pull to stretch the skin. Keep the stroke flowing in a smooth, even rhythm for several minutes.

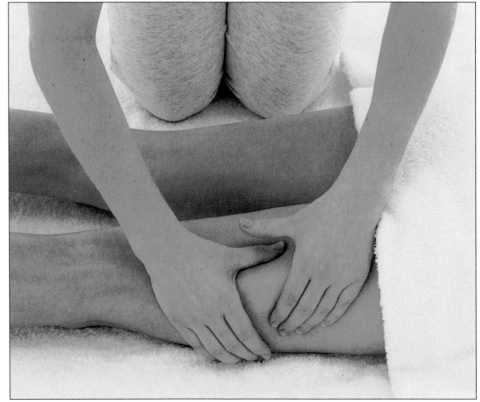

4 ▶ Stretch the back of the left leg again, by gently bending the heel up towards the bottom as far as is comfortable. Hold for a count of five, then release and repeat. Next, knead the back of the thigh muscle all over, using both hands to pinch the flesh between the thumbs and fingers as you press deeply into the muscle. Curve your fingers around the leg to knead the sides of the thigh; continue for several minutes. Finish off with two firm knee to thigh palm strokes, as in step three.

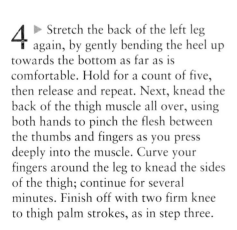

5 ▶ Still on the left leg, start with your hands on the calf above the ankle. Place them so that your wrists are together, with your fingers pointing down, wrapped around the leg. Press down into the heels of the hands with the fingers relaxed, then slide your hands out and away from each other around the leg. The movement is as if you are pushing the flesh in opposite directions, around to the front of the leg. Repeat, working up the calf, and stop just below the knee. Then continue above the knee, working up to the top of the thigh.

6 ▼ The person being massaged should turn face up. Bend her leg so that it is raised and tuck her foot between your knees. Wrap each hand, one above the other, around her ankle so that your thumbs are to the front and your fingers curve around the back. Push up from the ankle to the knee with a firm pressure, one hand following the other. At the top, fan out your hands and palm stroke firmly back down each side of the calf. Then grip round the ankle and repeat several times in a smooth motion.

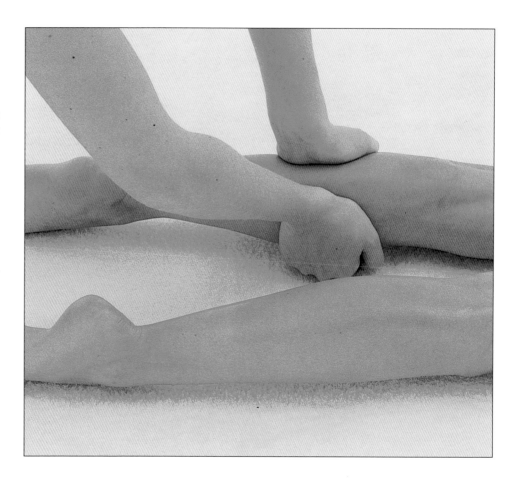

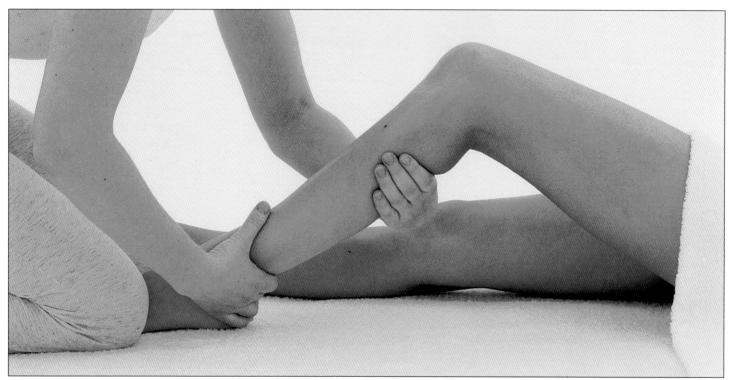

7 ▷ In the same position, move further forward so you can do the next stroke from the knee to the top of the thigh. With one hand palm up, place your thumb on the side of the thigh with your fingers wrapped around the back. With a firm inward pressure, slide your hand up the back of the thigh, then fan it round and do a palm stroke back down the front of the thigh. The hands should follow, one after the other, in a smooth, flowing motion so that each takes a turn to do the complete up and down stroke. Repeat for several minutes.

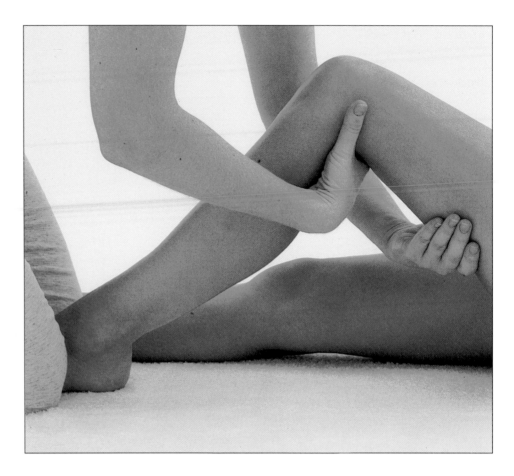

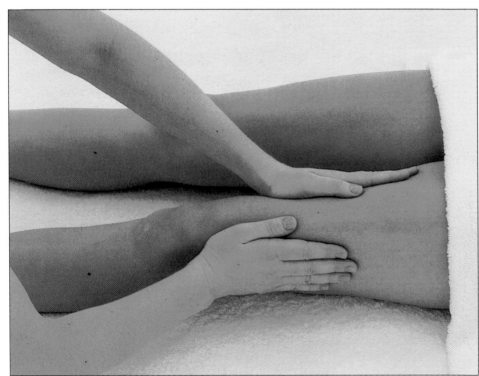

8 ◁ Straighten the leg and place one hand, palm down, on each side just above the ankle bone. With your hands working in unison in a backwards and forwards sawing motion, do a short, fast friction rub. Gradually move up the sides of the leg from ankle to thigh. Repeat from the ankle up again, this time bending the knee up so that you can rub the leg with one hand at the front and one at the back. Then do steps one to eight on the other leg in exactly the same way. Finish off by holding the legs firmly at the ankles and pulling them gently away from the body to extend them. Hold for a count of ten, release, then repeat.

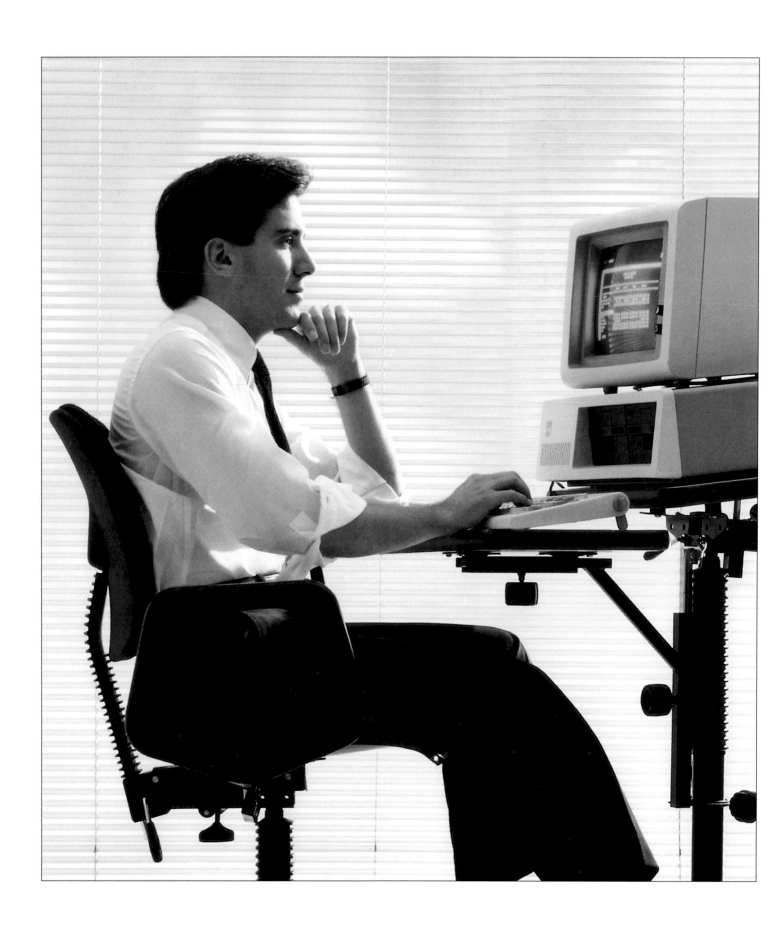

MASSAGE FOR ACHING HANDS OR WRISTS

This massage is a series of very simple stretches and strokes to help bring relief to hands that ache – whether as a result of tension or manual work. There is little real manipulation involved, just gentle flexes and finger strokes to release tension and soothe tender areas. It can, therefore, be used to relieve pain from almost any hand or wrist complaint, from too much knitting or tennis to rheumatism or arthritis.

The gentle, stretching movements are particularly helpful with Repetitive Strain Injury (RSI), one of the commonest new ailments of this decade. This affects people whose hands make the same movements repeatedly several times a minute, day after day – such as computer operators and factory workers – until the strain causes injury.

This massage is most useful in helping to prevent RSI occurring, so if you do a job that involves rapid, repeated hand movements, follow the routine once a day. Additionally, every 20 minutes on the job, try to take a brief break to shake your hands loosely in the air for a couple of minutes, then do the palm and wrist stretches from the first four steps of the massage. You can easily adapt them to do on yourself if you hold the side of the hand against your abdomen while you do the crosswise palm stretches in steps one and four. However, if you do have a job that you feel may be causing RSI, you should seek expert advice immediately.

HOW TO MASSAGE ACHING HANDS OR WRISTS

As this massage is meant for hands that ache, never take any of the stretches beyond the point of comfort – stop if the person you are massaging even so much as winces while you are extending his palms, wrists or fingers and immediately release the tension. For the same reason, keep the thumb strokes in steps five and six slow, light and gentle, so they are soothing rather than stimulating.

It helps to use lots of oil with this massage, not only because the skin on hands is naturally dry, but also because there are so many small bones and tendons close to the surface you need extra slip for comfort. If there is any inflammation of the hands, it also helps if you soak them in very warm water for ten minutes to boost circulation and soothe them before you start the massage.

(Left) Repetitive Strain Injury (RSI) can become chronic, forcing the sufferer to change jobs.

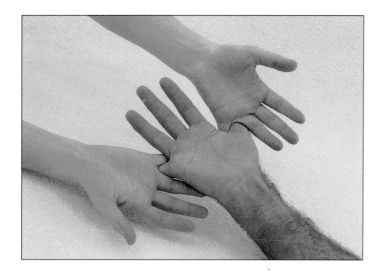

1 ◀ Do all steps on the right hand first, then repeat from the beginning on the left. Start with a simple palm stretch to release tension. Use the little and ring fingers of your left hand to grasp the thumb in a scissor-like hold, and those on your right hand to grasp the little finger. Once they are firmly interlocked, push down and out to stretch open the palm. Hold

2 ▶ Hold the right forearm of the person being massaged in the palm of one hand to support it, then interlock the stiff fingers of your other hand through his fingers so that they are criss-crossed. Gently push your hand up and back to stretch from wrist to fingertips. Only go as far as is comfortable so that you do not over extend the stretch, and push back from the tips of his fingers, not the base. Hold for a count of 15, then release.

3 Hold his right forearm, palm down, with your right hand to support it. Lay your palm over his knuckles, so that your fingers are pointing in the opposite direction to his. Gently push down with the heel of your hand into the first joint of his fingers close to the knuckles to flex the back of his hand. Hold for a count of 15, then release.

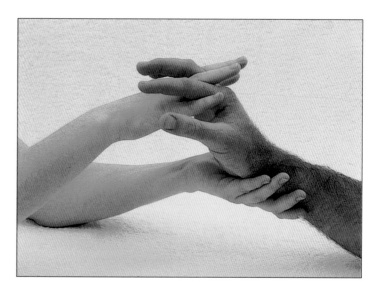

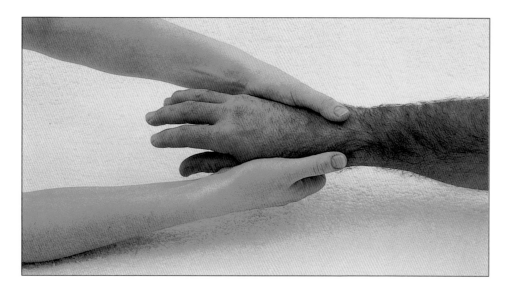

4 ◀ Place your wrists together and wrap your hands, palms down, around the back of his right hand with your fingers curved round to the front. Using the heels of your hands, slide them apart in opposite directions to roll his hand under and stretch it across the back. Hold for a count of five, then release and repeat.

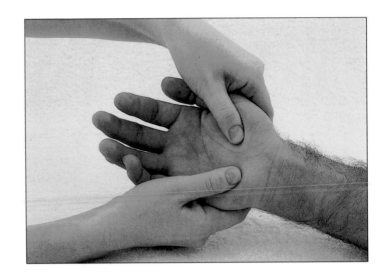

5 ▶ Tuck your fingers under the back of his hand and pick it up. Using your thumbs only, make small circles all over the palm of his hand without exerting any downward pressure. It should be a soothing stroke, not a kneading one, and very light so that your thumbs just glide over the skin. Finish off by using the sides of your thumbs to do long, straight palm strokes from wrist to fingers.

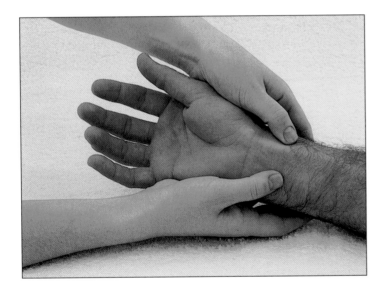

6 ◀ In the same position, slide your hands along until your thumbs are over the inner wrist. Then do very light strokes with your thumbs working in unison along each side of the tendon for about 5 cm (2 inches) before fanning them out to each side. Next, encircle the wrist with the thumb and first two fingers of your hands and do a light wringing motion, by moving one hand clockwise as the other goes anti-clockwise.

7 ▶ Hold the forearm of the person being massaged in the palm of your right hand. Slide the back of your left hand up under his palm, then push your fingers forward to interlock with his, and by pulling them back up toward you, lightly stroke between his fingers up to the nails. Keep repeating the whole palm to fingertip stroke in a smooth flowing motion. Finish by sandwiching his hand between your palms and lightly pressing for a count of ten.

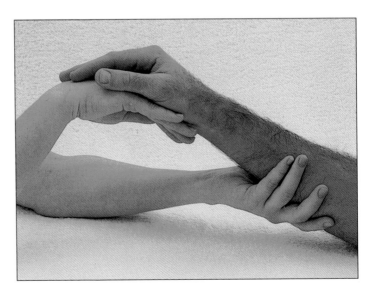

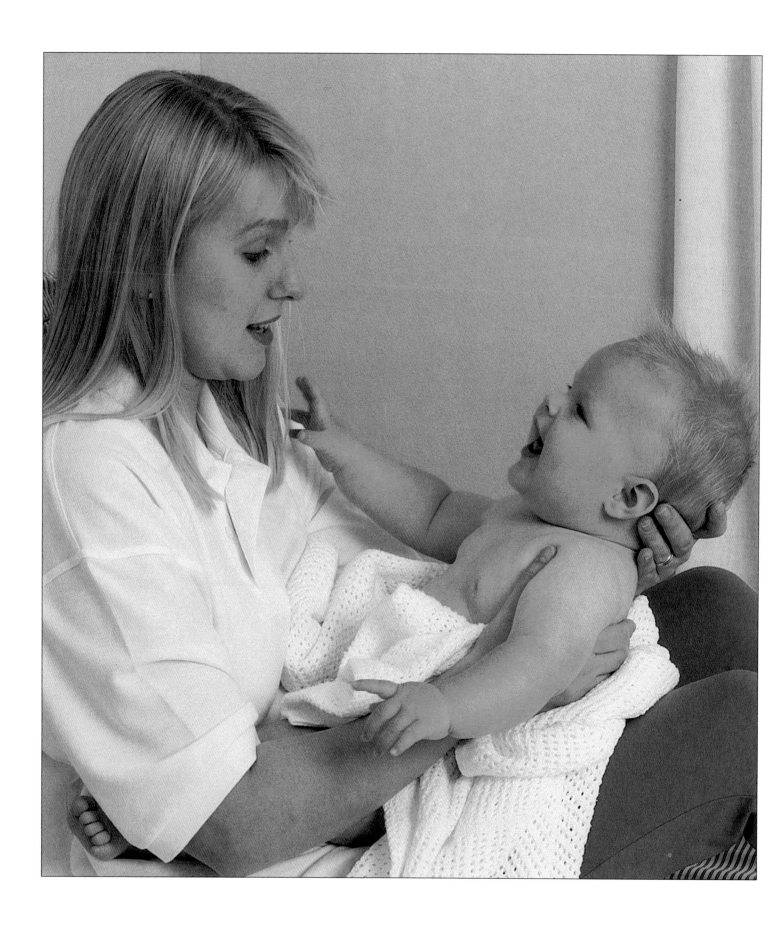

MASSAGE TO SOOTHE A RESTLESS BABY

Nothing is more stressful and irritating to even the most devoted parent than the constant cry of a baby. Although this massage works miracles, unfortunately it does not guarantee gurgles and smiles. In fact, it is best to practise this soothing massage when your baby is happy and relaxed. If you do it regularly from an early age, then the routine will calm the child before he starts roaring his little lungs out.

To being with, keep each step short and gradually increase the amount of time you spend on any parts he seems to enjoy. The massage uses slow, rhythmic stroking, with the emphasis on holding the baby close so he feels safe, snug and secure. It also gives you the chance to gaze into your baby's eyes and sing, talk, or just look at each other.

You can start this massage from four weeks old. Always be very careful not to use downward pressure with any of the movements – they should be light, skin strokes that hypnotically relax your baby. Remember it is the slip of the oil, the warmth of your hands, the smell of your skin, the sound of your voice and the rhythm of the movements themselves that work the magic, rather than the actual strokes.

HOW TO MASSAGE A RESTLESS BABY

To ensure that the baby feels comforted, snug and secure, always keep to the same routine until he is used to the massage. Straight after the morning or evening bath is an ideal time to rub in oil, although the stroking will put him to sleep immediately if he is already tired. Once he recognizes this as a special, cuddly routine – usually from ten weeks old – you may do it whenever you wish.

Make sure the heating is switched on and the room is cosy so that the baby can be bare without any harm. Nevertheless, you should also wrap areas of skin that are not being stroked in a blanket to keep them warm throughout. Have some tissues or old towels to hand – babies always go to the toilet as soon as you remove a nappy!

Finally, before you first do the massage, try out the most comfortable positions for steps five to eight – particularly if you have recently given birth and may be stiff or sore. If it helps, steps five and eight may be done sitting up on your knees, and steps six and seven may be done lying on your side.

(Left) The more soothing you are when massaging your baby, the more soothed baby will be.

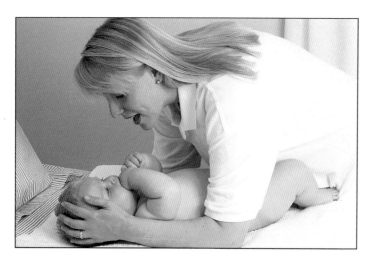

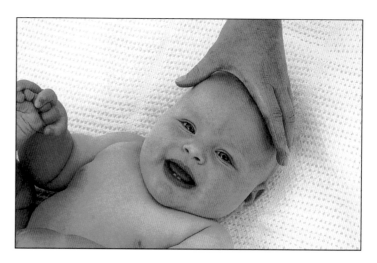

1 ▲ Before you oil your hands, kneel on the floor and bend forward over the baby, resting your arms on the bed on either side of the his body. Place your palms above his ears with your fingertips touching at the top of the head. Relax in this position so you are comfortable, but leave a gap between you. Gently cup the baby snugly so he feels secure, almost as if he were in the womb. Look into his eyes, smile or talk quietly. After a while, gently stroke from the forehead back to the crown in a rhythmic movement.

2 ▲ Rub a small amount of oil well into your hands, then gently place one hand across the top of the baby's forehead, with thumb on one side, fingers to the other. Gently stroke back over the head right to the crown. Repeat several times in a soothing, slow, light stroke that does not put any pressure on the baby's head. Place your palms around each side of his face and gently move them upwards to the top of the head. Repeat several times.

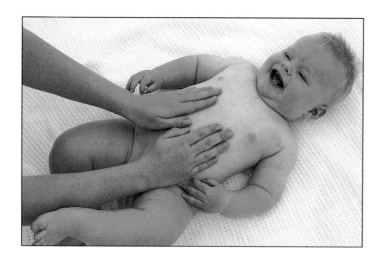

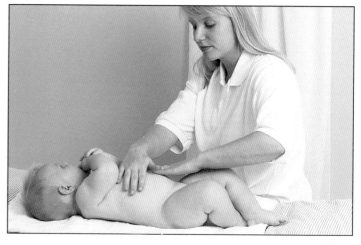

3 ▲ With a little more oil, place your hands on the baby's shoulders and stroke downwards over the chest, tummy, thighs, legs and feet. Repeat many times in a light, flowing rhythmic movement. Then place a cover over the lower half of the body for warmth and finish with a series of shoulder to tummy strokes, one hand after the other, in a continuous movement. Most children relax completely when their tummies are stroked and become so tranquil they hardly move at all.

4 ▲ Place your hand on the baby's abdomen between the ribs and, with the gentlest, lightest movement, make sweeping circles in a clockwise direction right around the navel. Use both hands, so that one finishes a circle as the other begins. Do not place any weight downwards at any time. Finish by stroking up and down the tummy with the palm of one hand in a rhythmic, soothing motion as lightly as possible.

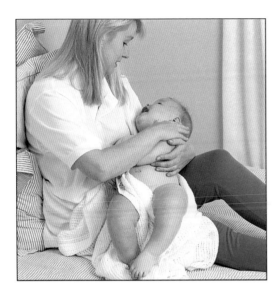

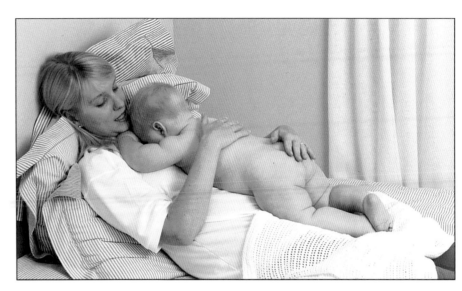

5 ▲ Now sit yourself comfortably on the bed and pick up the baby, cradling him side-on to your chest with one arm so his head is resting near your heart. Use your other arm to stroke gently down the side of the baby from head to foot. Start with you hand on his head and as you move down, use your wrist and inner arm as part of the stroke. Repeat several times, then swap arms and reverse the baby to stroke the other side.

6 ▲ Lean back so that you are comfortably propped against pillows and lay the baby face down against your chest. With more oil on your hands if needed, stroke from the shoulders down the back, over the bottom to the toes. Use a soothing sweep, with one hand starting as the other finishes for a continuous movement, so that you never lose skin-contact with the baby. Keep the same pace and rhythm going throughout and continue as long as you are both enjoying it.

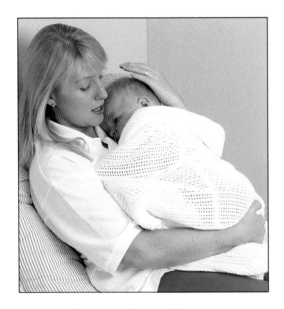

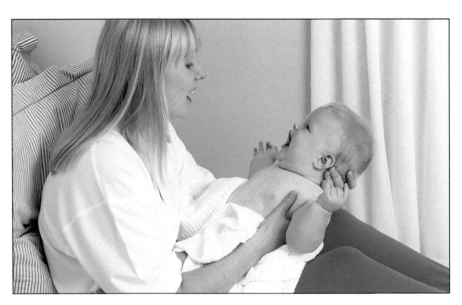

7 ▲ In the same position, place a warm cover over the baby and cuddle him to your chest with one hand. Use the other hand to cradle and gently stroke the baby's head from the top down to the nape of the neck. Again, keep a slow, soothing rhythm going throughout.

8 ▲ Finish off by sitting up slightly, bending your knees, and as you move the baby away from your chest, wrapping the cover right around him. Let the lower half of the baby's body slide down into your lap; support his head with one hand and his back with the other, so he is 'sitting' facing you. Enjoy some quiet time – look into the baby's eyes, sing, talk, kiss, cuddle or stroke his head if you wish.

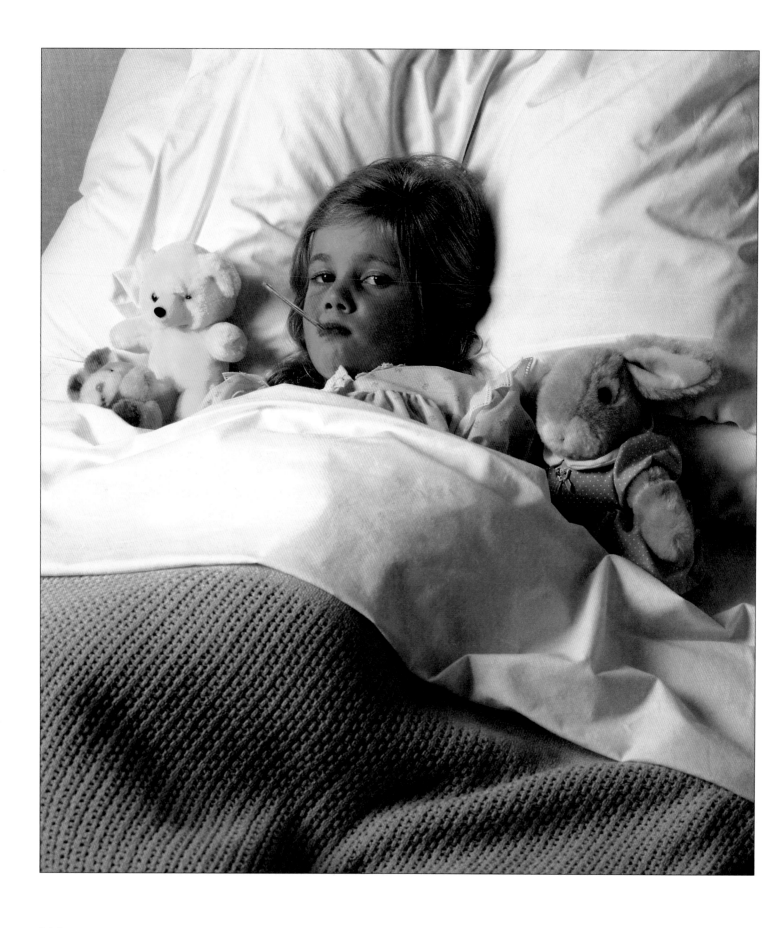

MASSAGE FOR A CHILD'S TUMMY ACHE

✳

Tummy ache is one of the commonest ailments of childhood. Little wonder when you see the quantities of food children can put away in no time at all, often without stopping to draw breath, let alone wait for anything to be digested. Although they seem to have cast iron constitutions, sometimes the average birthday party mix of lemonade, ice-cream, chocolate, sweets, crisps, cake and biscuits in one sitting has been known to cause a rebellion. More often than not, the pain starts at night, and the child cannot sleep, which makes it all seem much worse.

Massage works miracles on tummy ache. It helps soothe the pain, just the way rubbing a banged elbow or knocked knee does. The warmth, rhythm and touch of skin on skin have an almost hypnotically soothing effect on children. It is also a close, loving way to make a child feel better so that he goes back to sleep with sweet dreams.

When you stroke the tummy, always use the lightest, softest, slowest touch because not only is the abdomen sensitive, but it also responds best to gentle massage. Any strokes around the navel should always be done in a clockwise direction, as this aids the digestion of food and elimination of wastes.

If you child has persistent tummy aches, or the pain seems to get very much worse after three hours from the time it first appeared, seek medical advice as it may be something other than just an upset tummy.

HOW TO MASSAGE A CHILD'S TUMMY ACHE

The secret to curing tummy ache with massage is to keep movements simple, use lots of oil and do many repetitions. Once you have finished all six steps, put a warm hot water bottle on the tummy so the heat will keep the muscles relaxed. Do not massage a child's tummy immediately after a large meal – wait at least an hour – and do not do this massage on anyone under the age of two.

The best position for this massage is for you to sit at the child's side while he lies on a bed. If the child is very young, you may prefer to stand and bend low over him so that you can look into his eyes, sing or talk. He should lie comfortably on his back throughout, keeping his knees bent if the tummy muscles are tight or in spasm.

(Left) Children get tummy ache more than adults because their bodies are still growing.

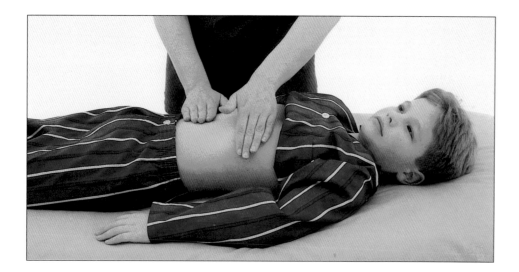

1 ◀ Sit at the side of the child's body. Place your right hand over the solar plexus and your left below the navel in the middle of the tummy. Make large, slow, sweeping circles in a clockwise direction around the abdomen, with the right hand moving down to the navel and the left hand moving up to the ribs. Repeat, so they do the same half-circle each, time and time again.

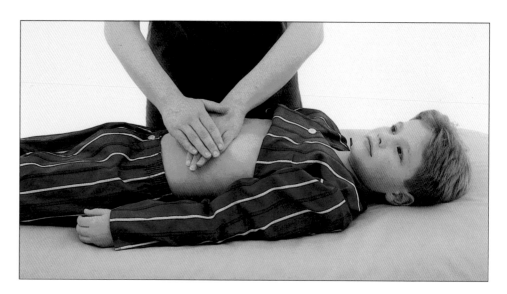

2 ▶ From the same start position, place one hand on top of the other, palms down, and make large clockwise circles around the abdomen – from the solar plexus, follow the ribs, then down across the groin and up the other side back to the start. Keep the movement light, rhythmic and soothing so that your hands make large, slow circles for several minutes.

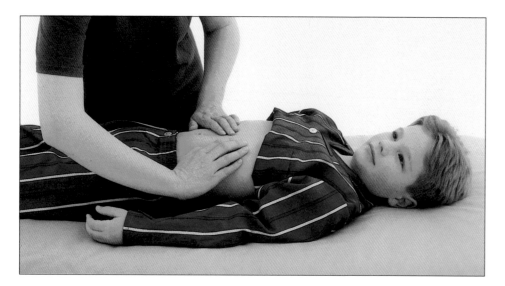

3 ◀ Place your hands, palms down, over the navel with your fingers covering the solar plexus at the base of the ribs. Leave them lightly resting there for a count of six, then slide them out to the sides, down the waist and round the lower abdomen. Then lift your hands and place them back in the start position and repeat the entire stroke for several minutes.

4 ▶ Now do some side stroking. Place your hands, palms down, over one hip with your fingers tucked under the bottom. Pull one hand after the other firmly up the body toward the abdomen, using your fingers to pull the flesh up and drag it back towards the tummy. Keep the stroke smooth, light and flowing so that it is pulling up and not pressing in. After several minutes, swap to the other side.

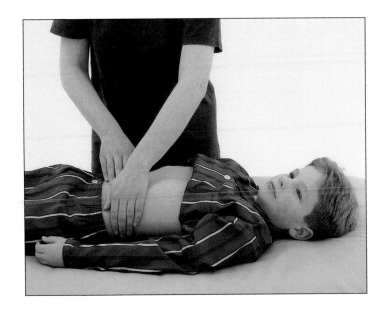

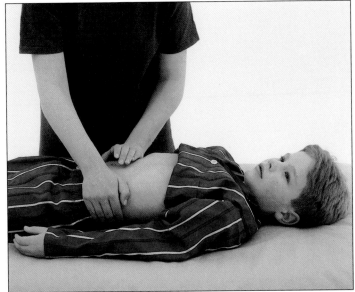

5 ◀ Do some cross-stroking over the entire tummy. Start with the fingers of the right hand tucked down under the back and the left hand resting across the tummy, both palms down. Pull up with your right hand, while the left glides across the tummy; as they cross, the left hand pushes down and the right glides lightly over the tummy without downward pressure. Repeat for several minutes.

6 ▶ Finish off with some slow, simple cat stroking. This is a light, flowing stroke with hands palms down, one following the other from the base of the ribs down the tummy to the groin. There should be minimal pressure, and as the lower hand reaches the end of the stroke, curve the palm so only the fingertips touch the skin. Make the stroke slower and gentler over several minutes, until you stop.

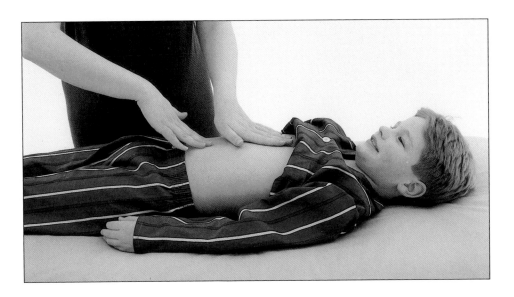

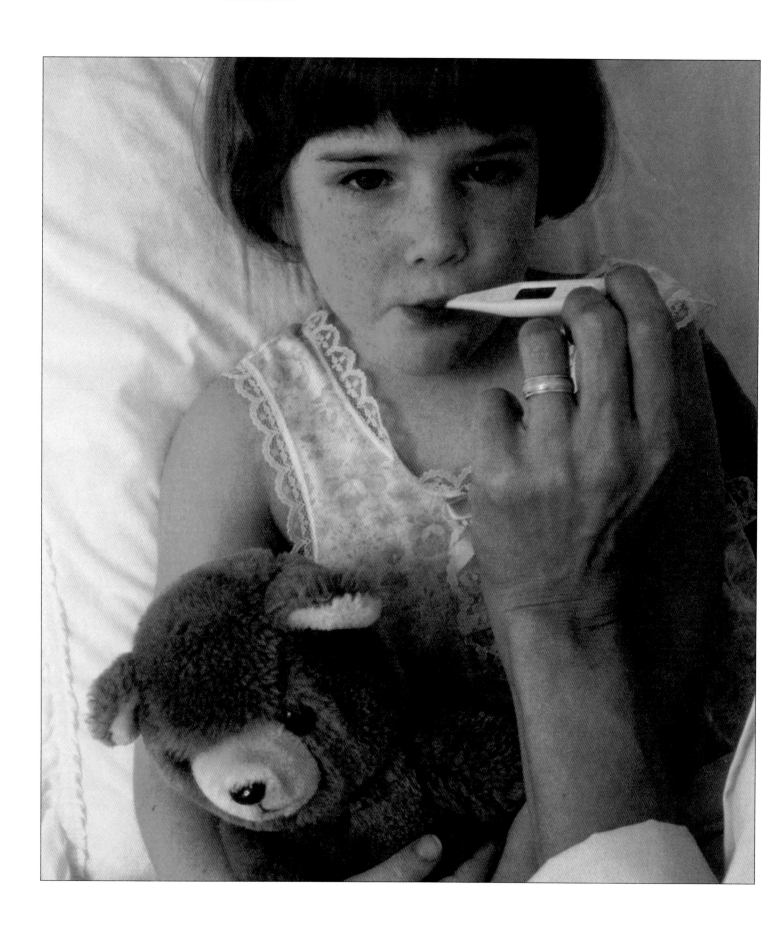

MASSAGE TO SOOTHE A CHESTY COUGH

Whether germs are getting stronger or we are getting weaker, the fact remains that hardly a family escapes a winter without at least one bout of sneezing and wheezing.

Although the common cold is relatively harmless, it can make you feel absolutely awful. This is particularly true when it goes to the chest when it makes you wheeze, mucus builds up in the nasal passages and you cannot breathe; then you start coughing and you cannot get a wink of sleep all night.

This massage helps in three ways. First, the slow stroking movements relieve any muscular aches in the chest caused by a persistent, hacking cough. Second, the tapping and light pummelling help dislodge congestion so it is more easily expectorated. Third, the warmth generated by stroking the chest and back help soothe the entire area and ease breathing.

This massage can be used for anyone of any age. For children, just do all the movements with much lighter hands than you would on adults. However, it is not recommended for asthmatics, anyone who suffers from chronic respiratory problems such as pneumonia, or anyone who has heart problems.

HOW TO MASSAGE TO SOOTHE A CHESTY COUGH OR COLD

You should do this massage after a bath and before bed. It is even more therapeutic if you mix some eucalyptus oil or a proprietary decongestant with your massage oil to help ease the breathing and stop the nose blocking in the night.

Warm the oil beforehand by standing the bottle in a basin of very hot water for ten minutes. If there is a lot of chest congestion, place two pillows under the lower back and waist so that the sufferer's head slopes downhill during the massage. The best positions for this massage are lying on a firm surface, face up for steps one to six and face down for the last two steps.

(Left) Constant coughs or colds throughout the winter seem to be a common complaint.

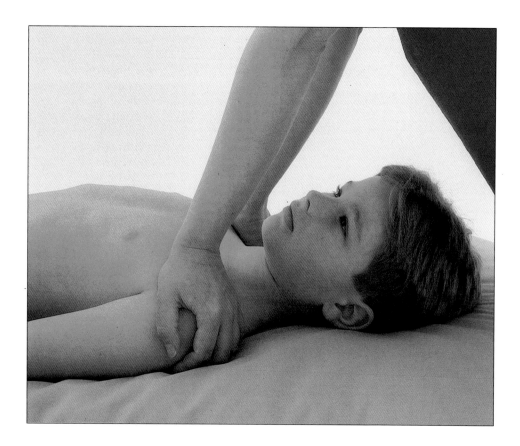

1 ◀ Steps one to six should be done with the sufferer lying on his back. Start by opening up the area: cross his arms over his chest, then lift up each one straight out to the sides at a 90° angle to the body. With arms back down at his sides, gently push down with the palms of each hand over the top of his shoulders. Hold for a count of seven, then relax. Then raise his arms up over his head and put them down beside each ear. Return the arms back to the sides.

2 ▶ Place your hands, palms down, across the sufferer's chest so that your fingers are touching over the breastbone. Glide your hands slowly apart and pull them back towards the armpits, around the top of the arms and back up over the shoulders to the start position. Repeat several times in one smooth flowing motion, with both hands working in unison towards each shoulder. It is a firm, slow, pulling stroke, but make sure your hands glide lightly over the collarbone.

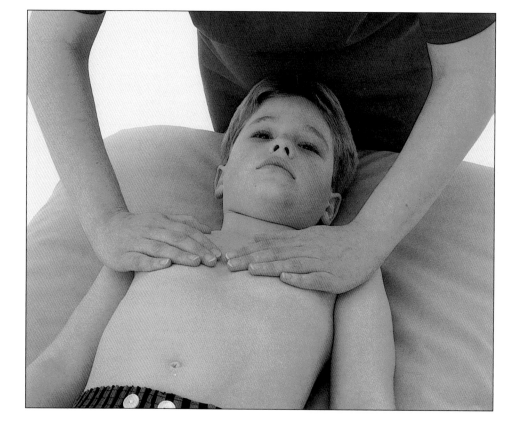

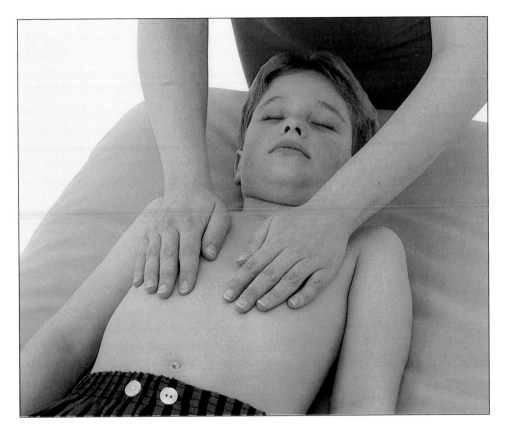

3 ◀ Place both hands, palms down, on the middle of the chest just below the collarbone, with your fingertips pointing towards the navel. Smoothly slide your hands down the middle of the chest, then fan them out, one to each side, over the bottom of the ribs. Pull back up the sides of the torso to the start position. Repeat as a slow, flowing movement for several minutes. The downward stroke should be light, with the upward one slightly firmer on the sides of the torso.

4 ▼ Place your left hand, palm down, flat on the upper chest below the collarbone. Make your right hand into a loose fist and use the base of the fist (heel of hand and little finger) to tap up and down on the back of the left hand. Use it like a hammer in a fast up-and-down bouncing movement that only raises the fist about 3 cm (1 inch). It should be a vibrating stroke, not a thump, to help shift chest congestion. Repeat every 5-10 cm (2-4 inches) all across the upper chest.

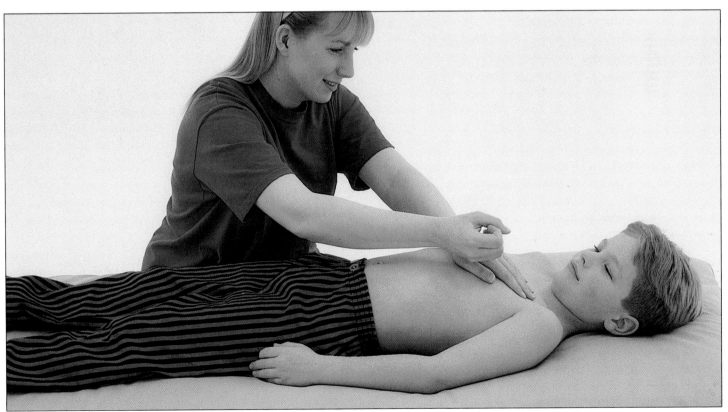

125

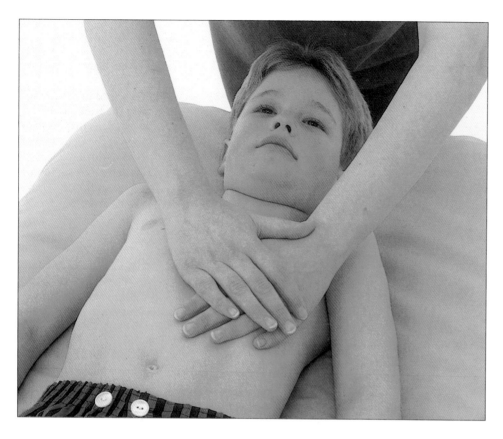

5 ◀ Place your hands, palms down and one on top of the other, in the middle of the chest where the ribcage parts. Use the top hand to guide the lower one and make large clockwise circles, working across the upper chest (the area between the collarbone and nipples). This is a stroke to push and sweep the skin – *do not press into the chest*. Try to continue long enough to generate heat between your hands and the sufferer's skin.

6 ▼ Now do a stretch to help open the chest area. Slide your hands, palms up, down under the sufferer's back so that your elbows are under his shoulders with one arm on either side of his spine. Take the strain by pressing down with your elbows as you turn your arms so that your hands are parallel, to make his back rise very slightly off the floor or bed. Hold for a count of ten, then relax. Aim to push the back up by an arm's width and not actually lift it, so the chest just spreads open at the front.

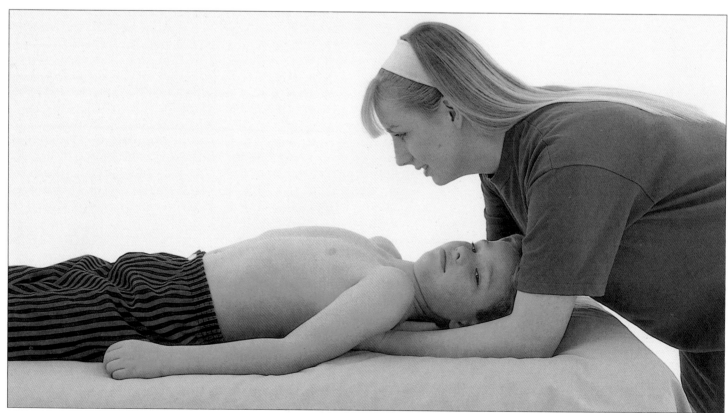

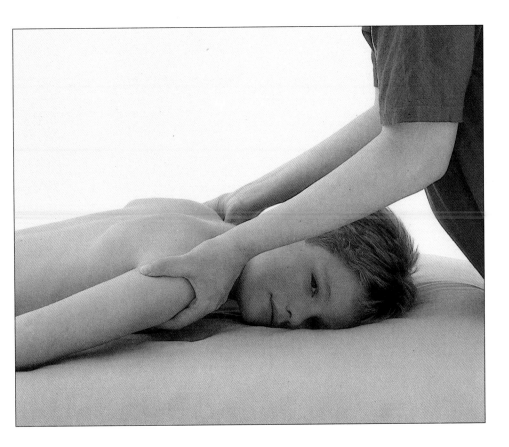

7 ◄ The person being massaged should turn over to lie face down for the rest of the massage. Place the palm of each hand around the top of each arm, with your fingers wrapped under to the front and thumbs on the back. Slowly pull both shoulders back so that they lift 5-10 cm (2-4 inches) off the floor or bed. Hold for a count of ten, then relax. Repeat step four, the vibrating palm-tap stroke, from the waist right up the back, avoiding both the spine and the bony shoulder blades.

8 ► Now do a 'pinky' flick all over the back. With your fingers straight but relaxed, use only the little fingers and the sides of your palms to flick the skin as you lightly bounce your hands up and down in a chopping movement. It should be fast, gentle and only 3-5 cm (1-2 inches) up and down, as one hand follows the other. Finish off by doing upward palm strokes from the waist to the tops of shoulders, with your hands working together on either side of the spine, and getting slower and lighter with each stroke.

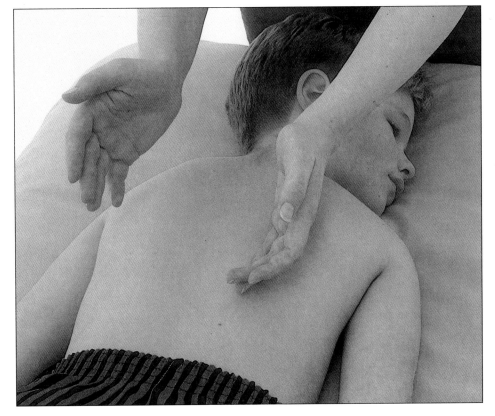

127

INDEX